Essentials of
Western
Veterinary
Acupuncture

Essentials of Western Veterinary Acupuncture

S. Lindley

and

T.M. Cummings

Blackwell
Publishing

© 2006 S. Lindley & T.M. Cummings

Editorial Offices:
Blackwell Publishing Ltd, 9600 Garsington Road, Oxford OX4 2DQ, UK
  Tel: +44 (0)1865 776868
Blackwell Publishing Professional, 2121 State Avenue, Ames, Iowa 50014-8300,
USA
  Tel: +1 515 292 0140
Blackwell Publishing Asia, 550 Swanston Street, Carlton, Victoria 3053,
Australia
  Tel: +61 (0)3 8359 1011

First published 2006 by Blackwell Publishing Ltd

ISBN-13: 978-14051-2990-9
ISBN-10: 1-4051-2990-5

Library of Congress Cataloging-in-Publication Data

Lindley, S. (Samantha)
    Essentials of western veterinary acupuncture / S. Lindley and T.M.
Cummings.
      p. cm.
    Includes bibliographical references and index.
    ISBN-13: 978-1-4051-2990-9 (pbk. : alk. paper)
    ISBN-10: 1-4051-2990-5 (pbk. : alk. paper)
    1. Veterinary acupuncture. I. Cummings, T. M. (Thomas Michael),
1963–. II. Title.
    SF914.5L56 2006
    636.089′5892–dc22

                                                          2005023986

A catalogue record for this title is available from the British Library

Set in 10/13pt Palatino
by SNP Best-set Typesetter Ltd., Hong Kong

For further information on Blackwell Publishing, visit our website:
www.BlackwellVet.com

Contents

Contents

Dedications

Preface

Sometimes it seems that in order to work in the field of veterinary acupuncture one must have the capacity to embrace and enjoy mystery. However, before the reader starts to edge nervously away from this text, it is worth pointing out that just because something is a mystery does not mean that it must be *mystical*. Similarly, just because there are limits to our understanding of a given technique there is not necessarily a limit to its efficacy. Recognising our current limits to understanding how the central nervous system works is probably all that is required to realise why we do not fully understand how acupuncture works. The central nervous system is amazing and complex enough without having to invent or look to explain further mysteries to illuminate the effects of acupuncture. Fortunately, in the rapidly developing world of neuroscience and neurophysiology some of the new discoveries indicate more clearly how the insertion of a needle into the body may inhibit pain and attenuate the signs of disease.

The field of pain research is rapidly expanding in human and veterinary medicine and revelations in this area tend to enhance our understanding of the use of acupuncture. It is both an exciting and a frustrating area in which to be involved; exciting because the outcome of research is fascinating and revealing; frustrating because the complete picture often seems further away with increasing knowledge of the vast complexity of the nervous system.

The promotion of a Western approach to veterinary acupuncture can also be frustrating because some of the veterinary profession are still highly sceptical, if not cynical, about the use of acupuncture. There are several likely reasons for this. First, acupuncture has been most often presented from a traditional Chinese medicine (TCM) approach. The vastly different language and diagnostic approach of this discipline sounds implausible to Western-trained minds and is therefore frequently dismissed as so much quackery. Second, there is limited evidence for efficacy of acupuncture in clinical conditions of the veterinary species. The reasons for this will become clear throughout this book. Third, whilst acupuncture continues to be regarded as 'alternative' to conventional treatment, there is likely to be an inherent resentment that orthodox thought and practice are being challenged.

However, it is not just the orthodox practitioners who may feel challenged. Among veterinarians, TCM has a small but enthusiastic following, part of which regards the Western approach as, at best, incomplete and, at worst, a misrepresentation of an ancient healing art. The Western veterinary or medical acupuncture practitioner may therefore feel somewhat between the devil and the deep blue sea.

We hope that this book will address some of these misgivings and help to place veterinary acupuncture firmly within the realms of orthodox veterinary practice. If its further use can be encouraged and research into its efficacy performed, then acupuncture has the potential to help alleviate suffering in more animals, which is, after all, the aim.

Samantha Lindley and Mike Cummings, 2005

About the authors

Samantha Lindley BVSc MRCVS

Samantha qualified from Bristol University Veterinary School in 1988 and, after a year's internship at Glasgow University Veterinary School, spent four years in mixed practice in Ayrshire. In 1993 she moved to Surrey where for four years she was veterinary behaviourist at Dr Roger Mugford's Animal Behaviour Centre. At this time, Samantha also ran a peripatetic acupuncture referral service in the Home Counties of England.

In 1997 Samantha moved back to Scotland and currently holds the position of Honorary Fellow at the Royal (Dick) School of Veterinary Studies, Edinburgh University, and Honorary Clinical Lecturer at Glasgow University Veterinary School. She runs behaviour clinics and acupuncture clinics at both veterinary schools and the Pain and Rehabilitation Clinic at Glasgow Veterinary School. Samantha writes and lectures extensively to veterinary undergraduates, veterinarians, veterinary nurses and welfare organisations on the subject of behaviour, acupuncture and pain management, clinically related behaviour problems and the welfare of captive wild animals.

Samantha has also developed and teaches an acupuncture course for veterinarians with Dr Mike Cummings, Medical Director of the British Medical Acupuncture Society (BMAS), and teaches acupuncture to medics at both basic and intermediate level on BMAS courses.

Samantha has acted as consultant to a variety of welfare organisations including Zoocheck Canada, WSPA Canada, Care for the Wild International, Animal Defenders, Born Free Foundation, Animal Aid, The Irish Society for the Prevention of Cruelty to Animals and The Dogs Trust. Samantha is the Honorary Veterinary Advisor to the

Captive Animal Protection Society and currently holds the position of Newsletter Editor and PR officer for the Association of British Veterinary Acupuncturists (ABVA).

Publications in non-peer-reviewed journals include articles on companion animal behaviour, reptile behaviour, complementary therapies and general welfare. Peer-reviewed articles include those on behaviour therapies, the results of work on the antiprolactin agent cabergoline, acupuncture, and reptile behaviour problems. Book chapters include a scientifically critical appraisal on complementary therapies for behaviour problems in the *British Small Animal Veterinary Association Manual of Canine and Feline Behaviour* (eds Heath, Horwitz and Mills, 2002); and two chapters in *The Con in Conservation* (ed. Dr Bill Jordan, 2001): 'Captive breeding' and 'Understanding human responses to endangered species'.

Dr Mike Cummings

Mike is Medical Director of the British Medical Acupuncture Society (BMAS). This is a full-time job that involves running the BMAS London Teaching Clinic (LTC), coordinating and lecturing on BMAS courses in Western medical acupuncture, acting as production editor for the Medline-listed journal *Acupuncture in Medicine*, and representing the BMAS at various academic and political meetings. He is an Honorary Clinical Specialist at the Royal London Homeopathic Hospital.

His principal academic and clinical interest is musculoskeletal pain, and in particular, needling therapies in the treatment of myofascial pain syndromes. He has completed a systematic review in this area.

He has been a member of the international editorial board for FACT (Focus on Alternative and Complementary Therapies) since August 1999. He is also a reviewer for *Annals of Internal Medicine*, *Archives of Physical Medicine and Rehabilitation*, the *British Medical Journal*, the *British Journal of Sports Medicine*, the *European Journal of Pain*, *Complementary Therapies in Medicine* and the *Journal of Alternative and Complementary Medicine*.

Contacts for the authors are through Samantha Lindley at s.lindley@dial.pipex.com c/o Glasgow University Veterinary School, Small Animal Hospital, Bearsden Road, Bearsden, Glasgow G61 1QH.

Introduction

WHAT THIS BOOK AIMS TO ACHIEVE

An understanding of Western veterinary acupuncture and the approach to treatment

There are already a number of texts aimed at the aspiring or practising veterinary acupuncture practitioner; however these tend to take either a predominantly traditional or a prescriptive approach, or both. In other words the rationale behind the treatment and selection of points described in these texts is based on the concepts of traditional Chinese medicine (TCM). This is a complex approach to both diagnosis and treatment and would have little or no meaning to the Western-trained veterinary surgeon. Some texts include formulae or prescriptions of points for given conditions: a sort of composite of the points likely to be chosen by a traditional practitioner. This satisfies neither the traditionalist (because each patient is an individual and is treated as such, as well as on how they present at any given time) nor the Western practitioner (because it means learning formulae or looking them up and does not take into account the results of examination and palpation of the patient), but has the merit of appearing both quick and easy.

This book aims to explain our current understanding of acupuncture from a neurophysiological perspective and therefore to help the practitioner work out which points to use, based on this understanding and on examination of the patient. This means that treatments *are* individualised, no formulae need be learned or looked up and the veterinarian can be satisfied that he or she is basing the treatment on the best available evidence.

A safe approach

Acupuncture is likely to be one of the safest interventions for the veterinary patient, aside from masterly inactivity on the part of the veterinarian. But acupuncture is not entirely safe. Reports of adverse events in humans are not uncommon and, although most are minor, some are fatal. There have been few official reports of problems in veterinary acupuncture practice, but this does not mean that they do not occur or that there is not the potential for them to occur. Safety issues will be discussed in this book, from safe positioning of the needle to cautions with and contraindications to needling.

A new understanding of muscular problems

Muscular pain is a significant cause of suffering in man and probably in mammals. Myofascial trigger points have long suffered from the Cinderella syndrome in orthopaedic/neurological and rheumatological considerations of pain and disease. This book aims to correct that and to encourage further study and the development of palpation skills by the reader.

A further understanding of pain

Veterinary acupuncture is most commonly used for the treatment of painful conditions. Understanding aspects of pain and how painful conditions may respond to acupuncture helps us to measure the effects of our interventions and assess whether or not we have alleviated suffering in our patients.

Some practical information

Once the reader is equipped with an understanding of acupuncture, the practical considerations of how to incorporate the technique into a clinic, frequency of treatment, restraint and handling techniques become relevant and are dealt with in Chapter 10.

Related techniques

There are devices and techniques that purport to act in the same way as acupuncture or that clients may propose to the veterinarian as having a likely benefit. The aim of Chapter 11 is to give a brief overview of these techniques, point the reader in the direction of more extensive information and suggest their likely relevance in the veterinary species.

WHO SHOULD READ THIS BOOK

Preparation for learning acupuncture

This book aims to go some way to help prepare veterinarians who are thinking about learning acupuncture. They may want some background knowledge or want to decide between courses that offer different approaches to the subject. However, it is *not* intended that this book will teach the needling technique to the veterinarian. Acupuncture is a practical technique that needs to be taught and practised under supervision. The palpation of skeletal muscle, essential for the identification of tender areas and myofascial trigger points, is a new skill for most veterinary practitioners and ideally should be demonstrated and experienced rather than visualised from text or images, however clear.

Enhancement of existing practice

It is hoped that this book will complement and progress the practice of those already practising acupuncture. It may also encourage a different approach by practitioners taught primarily by a TCM or a prescriptive route, or at least further an understanding of the Western veterinary/medical approach.

Researchers and research

Early indications of the best subjects for research often come from clinical observations in practice. It is in the interests of veterinary surgeons and our patients that we build up a reliable body of credible research in this field. This book may help to guide those involved in research in complementary and alternative medicine (CAM), but also encourage those in practice to keep records and carry out simple cohort studies to help highlight the areas that may be worth closer scrutiny.

Practitioners wishing to refer

Veterinarians in practice may have been approached by a veterinary acupuncture practitioner wishing to work locally or in the practice, or by clients requesting acupuncture for a variety of conditions in their pets. This book will help to explain how acupuncture works and how its likely efficacy for a given condition can be decided.

Veterinary nurses

As things currently stand, acupuncture is an act of veterinary surgery and therefore can only be legally carried out by a veterinary surgeon. It is possible however to train qualified veterinary nurses to perform acupuncture under direction from a veterinary surgeon suitably qualified to train them in the technique. In other words, veterinary nurses can act as technicians, placing the needles at the depth and position prescribed and previously decided by the veterinary surgeon, but cannot decide on alterations of treatment.

This book should provide a solid background of current understanding for veterinary nurses either trained in this capacity or wishing to be so.

Part One

Part One

Modern veterinary acupuncture

RENT STATUS OF VETERINARY ACUPUNCTURE IN UK
TERINARY PROFESSION AND WORLDWIDE

A DEFINITION OF ACUPUNCTURE

Acupuncture means many different things to many people. It may be a robust electrical stimulation via acupuncture needles or it may involve barely touching the subject; or it may be any kind of intervention between these two extremes. This is one of the difficulties in discussing acupuncture and whether it 'works'. One cannot just slot acupuncture into the same protocols as used to test a drug. With a drug there is a predetermined preparation, presentation and dose rate. Not only does the 'dose' of acupuncture vary widely between therapists, the response of the subject is also variable, depending on the state and make-up of its nervous system.

Therefore, before any further discussion, it is imperative that acupuncture is defined. Bearing in mind that the word 'acupuncture' comes from two Latin words: *acus* meaning needle, and *punctura*, to penetrate (or *pungere* from pricking, the origin seems uncertain) – it should at least involve a needle and skin penetration:

> *Insertion of a solid needle into the body for the purpose of therapy, disease prevention or maintenance of health*[1].

Note that the needle is solid and that it is fine. The use of a hypodermic needle may produce some of the effects of acupuncture, but it also creates more local trauma. One of the aims of acupuncture is to produce a maximal beneficial effect with minimum trauma to the tissues or body as a whole.

3

CURRENT STATUS OF VETERINARY ACUPUNCTURE IN UK VETERINARY PROFESSION AND WORLDWIDE

There are no firm figures for the numbers of veterinary practitioners who practise acupuncture in the UK or worldwide. This is mainly because any qualified veterinarian can practise acupuncture in the UK so long as they feel competent to do so. There is no acupuncture qualification recognised by the Royal College of Veterinary Surgeons in the UK and the responsibility for competency and safety rests with the practitioner. The qualification that has been longest in existence is the International Veterinary Acupuncture Society (IVAS) certification. This is granted after completion of a recognised course, an examination and a number of hours of seeing practice. It is maintained through Continuing Education (CE) points awarded to scientific meetings by the IVAS committee, thereby both encouraging further study and demonstrating that a given practitioner has made the effort to keep abreast of up-to-date information.

The Association of British Veterinary Acupuncturists (ABVA) was founded in 1989 by John Nicol MRCVS who, with his wife Margaret, kept the association running for ten years, aided by help of a small band of stalwart and enthusiastic general practitioners with an interest in promoting the use of acupuncture. In the last five years the Association has undergone some radical changes and, like any fledgling, has had a few flight problems since leaving the security of the nest that was so ably built for it. ABVA is now aiming to become a registered charity, with a non-veterinary chief executive and a board of trustees made up of practising veterinary surgeons (all of whom have other interests in practice). There is an education committee and the association runs scientific meetings and educational days 'to promote the understanding and use of acupuncture throughout the veterinary profession for the benefit of animals under our (collective) care'[2].

ABVA is still a relatively small group of 170 or so practitioners and by no means represents all of the veterinary surgeons practising acupuncture in the UK, although this is a situation it seeks to address. ABVA has run long modular courses comprising both Western neurophysiological theory and traditional Chinese medicine.

The ABVA is affiliated to the British Small Animal Veterinary Association (BSAVA) and as such takes advantage of the opportunities to run one of its scientific meetings as a satellite to BSAVA Congress.

The Western Veterinary Acupuncture Group (WVAG) is a virtual 'e-group' set up to support veterinarians who have attended the

Western Veterinary Acupuncture Course – a two-weekend course run by the authors of this book to teach veterinary acupuncture based entirely on neurophysiological principles following a conventional, orthodox diagnosis of disease. This course has to date trained around 120 veterinarians.

At the time of writing the WVAG has joined forces with the ABVA to run 4-day acupuncture courses on which it is hoped further courses can be based.

Most veterinary acupuncture is incorporated into general practice as an adjunct to conventional treatment. There are some practitioners who use acupuncture as part of an entirely 'alternative' approach along with other therapies such as homeopathy, chiropractic and herbal medicine. Few would practise acupuncture as a sole therapy, although there is no reason not to do so. However, acupuncture is not a panacea and it could be argued that the skills and experience of the veterinarian can be put to better use than when employed as a monotherapist.

With the already overcrowded veterinary undergraduate curriculum and continuing suspicion from many academic colleagues of all things purporting to be alternative, it is not surprising that the teaching of acupuncture in veterinary schools is not yet glimmering on the horizon. An increasing number of students are exposed to the technique in practice, however, and many show an interest when it is employed in the Pain and Rehabilitation Clinic at Glasgow University Veterinary School run by one of this book's authors (SL). Special study modules in Western medical acupuncture have been incorporated into medical undergraduate curricula and this book's other author (MC) ran such a module at Oxford Medical School.

Worldwide, acupuncture is taught and practised among veterinarians, but the emphasis is largely on the traditional Chinese medicine approach since many practitioners have learned from the IVAS system. There are national groups in many countries and IVAS holds an annual congress in different countries where the host group can support and organise such a meeting.

THE PUBLIC PERCEPTION OF ACUPUNCTURE

While potentially raising the collective blood pressure of the profession, the glut of veterinary and animal programmes shown on television has served to highlight a range of therapies available to owners for their pets. Having succeeded in never watching any of these programmes, these authors can only report being told that acupuncture treatment is regularly featured. Popular animal magazines and the general press also run stories, individual case reports and features on local veterinarians practising acupuncture. It would seem that all things complementary are good copy in the present climate. The ABVA receives numerous calls from members of the public either enquiring about acupuncture in general or wanting to find a veterinarian in their area who can treat their pet. Owners who have received acupuncture themselves are often keen to find similar treatment for their pet, whether or not they obtained relief from their own symptoms.

There are quirky regional differences in attitude that reflect the practice and acceptance of medical or traditional acupuncture in the local human population. Where owners are regularly exposed to friends and family being offered or seeking acupuncture treatment they are sanguine about the same treatment for their pets. Others react with surprise to learn that such a thing is practised on animals. It is not uncommon for healthy scepticism to exist among clients even when they have agreed to treatment. Much of this doubt is based on misunderstandings and common misconceptions about the treatment and how it works. It is still commonly asserted that acupuncture 'only works if you believe in it, so how can it work in animals?' Perhaps unsurprisingly, success in these cases produces the most enthusiastic of converts and the most satisfaction in the mind of the practitioner since there is less likelihood that the owners have imagined or willed the animal to get better. There are other reasons to make one more circumspect about the direct results of the needling, of which more anon, but the owner placebo effect is minimised in these circumstances.

The general public perception of acupuncture as a therapy is that it is safe. It is very safe in competent hands, but it is not entirely safe. In the authors' opinion this is one good reason why it should remain an act of veterinary surgery. The profession will, however, only maintain acupuncture in this status if they are perceived to be addressing safety issues seriously and it takes very little to knock public confidence in a given treatment or medication once the media machinery is grinding. While it would be counter-productive to overemphasise the potential dangers of acupuncture, especially since there is little evidence of such in the veterinary field, it is incumbent on veterinarians to fully explain the risks and possible side effects of any treatment. Awareness among the public of a degree of risk from the procedure would also make an individual owner more circumspect about accepting treatment from a non-veterinary acupuncturist or practitioner.

Another perception is that acupuncture is 'natural'. The perception of safety arises directly from this view – i.e. that nothing natural can possibly be harmful. This is clearly not the case and, even if it were, there is nothing natural about sticking pointed bits of metal into the body, even if it has been done for hundreds of years. If pressed on this concept, it is likely that the true perception is that the effect is natural, rather than the intervention itself. In other words: the body's 'natural' balance is restored by acupuncture. To an extent this is true and will be discussed later. Unfortunately, such language conjures up images of floating kaftans and wafting incense, but acupuncture affects the nervous system more prosaically than mystically by acting as an unusual stimulus. The results of the stimulus are not unusual in themselves, because most natural systems will return to a set point if allowed to do so and the mammalian body has myriad checks and balances to achieve optimum functioning and, ultimately, survival.

Many clients are dubious about how well their pet will accept acupuncture. This is especially the case for cat owners, but many cats in fact tolerate the treatment remarkably well. Of course, there is always a degree of patient (and client) selection in any intervention, but most animals accept the treatment and some even appear to make positive associations with their visit to the pain clinic. Because there is no indication of distress, owners are more willing to persist with the treatment and make regular return visits.

In terms of effectiveness, the balance appears to be on the side of pleasant surprise when the acupuncture appears to work for their pet. There are a few owners who appear determined that the therapy will work come what may. In fact, in the author's experience (SL), these are the ones who seem most frequently disappointed. It is a difficult concept to grasp that their particular pet may not respond to this particular intervention. After all, the same treatment for the same condition should yield the same result if it is effective, should it not? In the numbers game it should, but even accepted treatments such as non-steroidal anti-inflammatory drugs (NSAIDs) do not work for every individual. Of course, when the result is a positive one, the credit is almost always given to the acupuncture even if there are concurrent therapies. This is because it is an unusual approach, because there is a physical interaction and an intervention that makes a strong visual impact on the owner. As veterinarians we tend to have more physical contact more regularly with our patients than do our medical colleagues, but there is still a strong appreciation of therapies that involve a sort of 'laying on of hands'. It is also the case that, because of palpation techniques that focus on the tenderness in muscle, pain can be elicited even in the most stoical of animals and this helps to convince owners that the veterinarian is close to the source of the problem.

During the course of acupuncture treatment it is often the practice to leave the needles in place for a variable amount of time. Communication between client and veterinarian at this time can enhance the history, but also the loyalty between therapist and owner and is therefore positive for the image of the individual, the practice and the profession.

SAFETY

Acupuncture is perceived to be a safe technique, both by the public and by some acupuncture practitioners. Although it is one of the safest interventions veterinarians are ever likely to make, it is not completely safe. This carries several implications:

(1) There should be responsible, and preferably centralised, recording of adverse reactions and side effects to acupuncture treatment delivered by veterinarians.
(2) Arguably, acupuncture should remain as an act of veterinary surgery so that animal welfare can be protected and so that there is a greater likelihood of recording adverse events.
(3) At some level, research should establish the specific efficacy of needle penetration. There are likely to be many non-specific effects of acupuncture that could be brought about without needle penetration. Since the risk arises when the needle penetrates the skin then that risk should be demonstrated to be necessary. Specific efficacy has been demonstrated in recent trials in medical acupuncture[3-6]. Because of ethical considerations it is problematic to conduct clinical trials to demonstrate this specific effect in veterinary conditions. Pragmatic outcomes such as comparing acupuncture with the recognised standard treatment are more workable and fit ethical guidelines (the protocol for a clinical trial must show intention to treat). However, it could be argued that, since human patients are likely to be more susceptible to placebo and non-specific effects, demonstration of the specific effect in this species may be sufficient to convince sceptics in the veterinary field.

There are few recorded cases of safety issues in animals:

(1) Three cases of silicone granuloma in horses[7]. Silicone coating is used in surgical, hypodermic and some acupuncture needles to ease skin penetration. In some individuals silicone oil deposits in the skin at puncture sites and sets up a foreign body, granulomatous type reaction. This phenomenon has been recorded in one person[8], and only in these three horses and so does not appear to be a significant problem, or a rational basis for changing the coating of needles.

(2) One case of deep abscess formation in the gluteal region of a dachshund (personal communication with SL). This is unusual. The skin is not swabbed in veterinary (or human) acupuncture and the area is not shaved. There is no attempt at aseptic technique, but the area should be clinically clean. In general terms the rule of thumb is that the patient's own flora is safe and the numbers of potential pathogens carried subcutaneously with the needle minimal. This is not the case if the patient is immuno-suppressed or if the area is contaminated with 'foreign' dirt such as mud, faeces or if the needle penetrates an area of the skin that is already infected. This is more likely to happen in the veterinary species since the skin cannot always be seen clearly.

In practice, there are occasional incidences of minor bleeding at some puncture sites. Bruising is likely, but is not an aesthetic problem with animals and is difficult to see. Since it may add minor discomfort to the existing condition it should be minimised.

Some animals are reported to sleep for extended periods of time following acupuncture (up to 24 h or even a week reported). This is not a problem in itself and would usually indicate a positive response to needling, but owners may be alarmed at this response when it first occurs. Most are delighted once they realise it is harmless since it indicates that something 'real' has happened.

Potential safety problems

These conditions have not been reported in the veterinary species following needling, but should be considered since there is no reason to suppose they should be exclusive to human acupuncture practice.

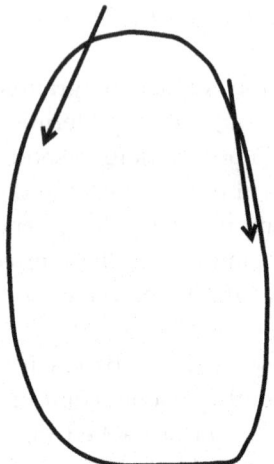

Figure 1.1 Cross section of canine thorax. Arrows indicate the direction of needling to avoid piercing the pleura.

Pneumothorax

Pnemothorax is the most frequently recorded serious and potentially fatal condition in humans following acupuncture over the thorax[9]. Although the needles are fine, it is presumed that on occasion they puncture a bleb formation or bulla on the lung giving rise to tension pneumothorax[10].

Since many acupuncture and trigger points are located over the thorax in the veterinary species it would seem sensible, if not imperative, to take a responsible approach to avoiding needling the lung and pleura. These will be reiterated later, but include:

- Needle at a tangent to the rib cage as shown in Figure 1.1. This is easier in most veterinary species because of their shape of the rib cage compared with that of a human.
- Needle superficially.
- Needle over a rib.

It is likely that there is a lower incidence of bullae in the veterinary species and it may be that the mediastinum may protect to a degree from bilateral pneumothorax, although in dogs and cats it is incomplete and the condition is likely to become bilateral anyway[11].

Scepticaemia

Incidences of scepticaemia have occurred in immunosuppresed human patients. Caution is advised if treating patients already receiving chemotherapy, those that are diabetic or with other conditions that may impair immunity.

Bleeding disorders

Coagulopathies, bleeding disorders, spontaneous bruising, von Willebrand's disease, and autoimmune haemolytic anaemia etc., are conditions in which needling cautiously is called for, especially in closed fascial compartments. Uncontrolled bleeding in these regions may cause compartment syndrome.

Neuropathy

Three cases of neuropathy secondary to acupuncture have been reported in humans[12,13], although there are probably many unreported cases of transient neuropathy. In one of the described cases a median nerve neuropathy was caused by a needle fragment in the carpal tunnel following accidental fracture of the needle. The fragment was removed at surgery. A second report describes two cases of peroneal nerve palsy resulting in foot drop, one of which resulted from acupuncture needling. There is no reason why such accidental fracture would not occur in the veterinary species and any unexplained neuropathies should be considered in the light of recent acupuncture therapy.

Pregnancy

Much is written and spoken about the wisdom of using acupuncture in pregnancy. In traditional Chinese medicine there are 'forbidden points'. These are to be avoided during pregnancy, because they can supposedly cause miscarriage and abortion in women. There is no evidence for this and the reluctance on the part of some human practitioners to use acupuncture during pregnancy is mainly for medico-legal reasons, i.e. miscarriage is common in the first trimester of pregnancy and the practitioner may be blamed for any such spontaneous events following needling. The same is probably true of the veterinary species: valuable brood mares and whelping bitches should be treated with caution, not because of a likelihood of causing a problem, but because of the likelihood of being blamed for a spontaneous event.

Local conditions

Acupuncture needles should not be inserted through areas of local infection, ulceration, oedema (because there is an increased risk of infection) or into anaesthetic areas (because the acupuncture will not work). Tumours should also be avoided.

Demand pacemakers

Increasing numbers of canine patients are fitted with pacemakers. If electroacupuncture is to be used in these patients the veterinarian should consult the cardiologist involved, but should in any case avoid connecting up and passing a current across the animal's chest (see: Chapter 11).

Potential interactions

There is no evidence to suggest that concurrent therapy of any sort will reduce the effects of acupuncture (see: Chapter 10). It has been claimed by some that non-steroidal anti-inflammatory drugs and corticosteroids somehow 'block' the effects, but there is no need to withdraw medication from animals before they receive acupuncture. The only caution with corticosteroids is to consider the length of treatment and dose because of possible detrimental effects on the immune system (see: Scepticaemia, above).

Other interactions

Needling in an area locally anaesthetised is pointless. Acupuncture requires an intact nervous system to work and local anaesthetic will stop the transmission of nerve impulses.

Needling under general anaesthesia may still be useful, especially for the treatment of trigger points, which can be palpated when the patient is anaesthetised. However, deep anaesthesia may block some of the other effects of acupuncture, so unless specifically treating active trigger points, it is probably better to use sedation if trying to acupuncture fractious or restless animals, or to acupuncture as the anaesthesia lightens postoperatively.

Symptomatic treatment

Acupuncture may give potent symptomatic control. It is therefore important, where possible, to establish a diagnosis before needling to avoid masking the signs of serious disease and delaying diagnosis. Some owners see acupuncture as a way of avoiding costly or involved diagnostic procedures.

Position of needles

Animals frequently lie down during acupuncture treatment. Placing needles ventrally will either require that the animal be safely restrained, so that the needles cannot penetrate into abdomen or thorax, or that needling is kept brief and the needles not left in place.

Common minor adverse events

(1) *Syncope*: Fainting is not uncommon in human subjects, but is not reported following needling in animals. The possibility of an anoxic 'fit' (as well as physical injury) is a risk in humans if they faint while sitting up or in a position where slumping will block the airways. One of the authors (SL) has witnessed a horse nearly collapse and then recover when a point in the cranial tibial muscle was needled. This event was repeated when the bilateral point was needled ten minutes later. The potential dangers here would be physical injury to the horse and to the handlers and considerable surprise to the veterinarian.

(2) *Sweating*: This occurs commonly in horses during or after acupuncture. It is not a problem in itself, but patchy sweating is often associated with painful conditions such as colic and may alarm an observant owner.

(3) *Pain*: Unpleasant pain can occur during needling, but ideally should be minimised. It may result from excessive stimulation of certain structures (skin, periosteum, fascial layers, ligaments, tendons, blood vessels or nerves) or from muscle spasm around the needle. Pain can persist after needling, but usually settles within a couple hours, or at most a few days. Very rarely postneedling pain can persist for much longer. This has been reported in humans rather than animals: in one case for a year after needling the first dorsal interosseous muscle (LI4) (White 1995, personal communication).

(4) *Stuck needle*: Needles often feel as though they are being 'gripped' by the muscles into which they are inserted. This grip usually relaxes during the treatment, but occasionally the needle is so firmly grasped that it cannot be withdrawn. In these rare cases it is possible to slide another needle in close to the first and then withdraw both.

(5) *Needle problems*: Needles can break, although this is less common these days because single-use, disposable needles are usually used. If needles are going to break then it is most likely to be at the junction of handle and shaft. Therefore, it is not good practice to insert needles up to the hilt, because, if fracture occurs, there will be no portion of needle left above the skin to grasp and remove. Other possible problems include: bending of needles from strong muscle contraction or clumsy handling and blunting or hooking of the needle tip resulting from multiple insertions or periosteal pecking. It is very common to remove needles that are twisted into coils from horses' backs, but this does not usually cause a problem apart from the alarm when it first occurs.

Auricular acupuncture-safety aspects

The insertion of needles into animals' ears with the intention of having a therapeutic effect is carried out by some veterinary practitioners. Apart from the potential practical difficulties and tolerance of this procedure, the use of stay needles (tiny needles shaped like tacks, designed to stay in the skin and kept in place by plaster) gives rise to two major risks. The first is that if the needles fall out then they can cause injury to an animal or human and the second is that the ear cartilage commonly becomes infected.

REGULATION

Currently, acupuncture for animals is an act of veterinary surgery. In the UK only a qualified veterinary surgeon can carry out acupuncture. A qualified veterinary nurse may needle under direction from a veterinary surgeon, provided they have received sufficient training. Although physiotherapists may have been trained to use acupuncture during their physiotherapy training they are not legally allowed to acupuncture animals, even if the animal has been referred to them for physiotherapy and they regard acupuncture as part of that discipline. There is new regulation concerning acupuncture on humans being drafted at the time of writing and it is uncertain as to how or whether it will affect veterinary acupuncture. It may be that the term 'acupuncturist' will become a protected title and its use limited to practitioners who have undergone specified training. This text therefore avoids using the term wherever possible.

THE FUTURE

(1) If it can be shown that acupuncture can have a beneficial effect on common veterinary conditions then it is possible that 'somatic sensory stimulation' will be taught in veterinary schools in the future.

(2) Research will demonstrate a specific effect of needling and will elucidate the mechanisms of acupuncture in treating chronic pain and non-painful, functional disorders.

(3) Acupuncture will become another in the growing array of tools to treat pain and alleviate signs of disease in the veterinary species.

Even if this utopian view is not realised, it is hoped that the study of and interest in acupuncture will promote further understanding about pain and pain perception in animals.

REFERENCES

1. Acupuncture Regulatory Working Group. *The Statutory Regulation of the Acupuncture Profession – The Report of the Acupuncture Regulatory Working Group*. The Prince of Wales's Foundation for Integrated Health; 2003. ISBN 0953945375

2. *Constitution of the Association of British Veterinary Acupuncturists*. Surrey, UK: ABVA; 1989.

3. Lee A, Done ML. The use of nonpharmacologic techniques to prevent postoperative nausea and vomiting: a meta-analysis. *Anesth Analg* 1999;88(6):1362–9.

4. Vas J, Mendez C, Perea-Milla E, Vega E, Panadero MD, Leon JM, Borge MA, Gaspar O, Sanchez-Rodriguez F, Aguilar I, Jurado R. Acupuncture as a complementary therapy to the pharmacological treatment of osteoarthritis of the knee: randomised controlled trial. *BMJ* 2004;329(7476):1216.

5. Berman BM, Lao L, Langenberg P, Lee WL, Gilpin AM, Hochberg MC. Effectiveness of acupuncture as adjunctive therapy in osteoarthritis of

the knee: a randomized, controlled trial. *Ann Intern Med* 2004; 141(12):901–10.

6. Witt C, Brinkhaus B, Jena S, Linde K, Streng A, Wagenpfeil S, Hummelsberger J, Walther HU, Melchart D, Willich SN. Acupuncture in patients with osteoarthritis of the knee: a randomised trial. *Lancet* 2005;366(9480):136–43.

7. Slovis NM, Watson JL, Affolter VK, Stannard AA. Injection site eosinophilic granulomas and collagenolysis in 3 horses. *J Vet Intern Med* 1999;13(6):606–12.

8. Yanagihara M, Fujii T, Wakamatu N, Ishizaki H, Takehara T, Nawate K. Silicone granuloma on the entry points of acupuncture, venepuncture and surgical needles. *J Cutan Pathol* 2000;27(6):301–5.

9. Rampes H, Peuker E. Adverse effects of acupuncture. In: Ernst E, White A, editors. *Acupuncture – A Scientific Appraisal.* Oxford: Butterworth Heinemann; 1999. pp. 128–52.

10. Peuker E. Case report of tension pneumothorax related to acupuncture. *Acupunct Med* 2004;22(1):40–3.

11. Evans HE. The respiratory system. In: Evans HE, editor. *Miller's Anatomy of the Dog.* Philadelphia: WB Saunders; 1993. pp. 483–93.

12. Southworth SR, Hartwig RH. Foreign body in the median nerve: a complication of acupuncture. *J Hand Surg [Br]* 1990;15(1):111–12.

13. Sobel E, Huang EY, Wieting CB. Drop foot as a complication of acupuncture injury and intragluteal injection. *J Am Podiatr Med Assoc* 1997; 87(2):52–9.

An historical perspective

TRADITIONAL CHINESE MEDICINE (TCM) – AN OVERVIEW

Acupuncture and acupuncture-like stimuli have been in evidence for thousands of years. It would seem that when any group of people live together and live long enough to develop muscle strain and the 'luxury' of chronic pain (for one must be alive to feel chronic pain) that comes with injury and degeneration, they find increasingly ingenious ways of alleviating their discomfort.

From simple rubbing where it hurts to providing a potent distraction in another area of the body, man has discovered empirically that physical interaction with the body can have therapeutic effects. It does not take a great leap of imagination to visualise that from rubbing a muscle one may progress to getting someone else to rub it or to put pressure on that tender area. Once rocks were employed as implements to help in other tasks it is logical to assume that man learned to use such crude tools to achieve greater or more intense pressure on a given area of the body. It would have been realised, if not described in these terms, that the smaller the surface area of an implement the more intense the stimulus and the more effective it was in relieving the pain.

The evidence for acupuncture as a common technique

From historical documents it is clear that acupuncture and acupuncture-like stimuli have developed all over the world in cultures whose peoples had no cultural crossover. In other words the technique was not always 'spread' by demonstration or description, but arose probably as described above: from simple methods that had been observed to help pain and perhaps other forms of disease.

For example: the Papyrus Ebers are an Ancient Egyptian medical treatise and these describe the use of acupuncture-like treatments, as do the Vedas, which are the most ancient scriptures of Hinduism. The Vedas were not written down until about 1300 BC, but were passed down through the generations by word of mouth. These scriptures are thought to be 5000 to 7000 years old and contained within them is the Ayurveda, or 'Science of life', which includes reference to the use of acupuncture.

In 1991 the frozen remains of a man were discovered in the Similaun Glacier of the Tyrolean Alps. The body had been undisturbed for over 5000 years. This remarkably well-preserved 'Iceman' (named Ötzi) sparked much debate, including border arguments over whether he belonged to the Italians or the Austrians. The investigation into Ötzi's demise must have the record for being the oldest murder enquiry, until forensic evidence showed that he had probably been killed in a skirmish. Ötzi's body also showed evidence of a skin piercing technique, probably very similar to a developing form of acupuncture[1,2]. This would date the use of acupuncture-like stimuli in Central Europe to around 3200 BC. Animals began to be domesticated in China between the sixteenth and seventeenth centuries BC and at this time it seemed that practitioners of medicine would treat both animals and people. But from the Zhou Dynasty (1122–770 BC) onwards the disciplines appeared to separate and the first written description of a distinctly veterinary approach was by Bai-Le in 650 BC in Bai-Le's Canon of Veterinary Medicine, although whether Bai-Le actually existed as a person is in some contention.

The earliest acupuncture instruments reflected the materials to hand and the skill of the culture employing them in the way that they were shaped into appropriate forms. Very early instruments were made from sharpened stone ('bian'), and there followed a progression of needle-like implements fashioned from bone, bamboo, copper, iron, silver, gold and finally stainless steel, the latter being most commonly used in modern practice. Early implements were not fine or sharp enough to penetrate the skin easily so some early descriptions of acupuncture paint vivid pictures of small hammers being used to drive the 'needle' into the body[3].

There are a number of legends and apocryphal stories from China describing how acupuncture was first developed. One of the most commonly repeated tales describes observations on the battlefield: soldiers who were pierced by arrows in certain parts of the body had other symptoms relieved or diseases elsewhere in the body cured. Similar stories have been told about horses suddenly becoming sound in another limb or being cured of disease after being wounded by arrows. It seems likely that the truth is more prosaic: rather than being as a result of dramatic enlightenment on the battlefield, acupuncture probably developed slowly from observation of what humans do to themselves and each other when something hurts: rub it better, massage, pressure, distraction!

Traditional Chinese medicine

Whatever else may have been happening throughout the world for hundreds of years, it was the Chinese who developed a complex system of medicine that incorporated acupuncture, but did not use it exclusively, and who formalised this system and described it in detail. With the addition of other ideas and techniques from India, the system then spread to other cultures.

It is not within the remit of this book to discuss traditional Chinese medicine in detail, but those exploring acupuncture outside these pages will inevitably be exposed to the ideas and concepts. It is therefore worth putting it into context.

Traditional Chinese medicine is a diagnostic as well as a therapeutic discipline. It is highly complex and involves ideas and concepts that have been added to the existing ideas, e.g. the 'Five Phases' were probably derived from India. This practice of incorporating other ideas into the system is known as syncretism and tends to keep systems and practitioners together, rather than encouraging them to break away into sects following their own beliefs and practices.

TCM developed around the use of acupuncture and herbal remedies. As it developed, the system was influenced by a number of the prevalent philosophies. The main influence came from Taoism (pronounced *Daoism*). Laotse (circa 500 BC) is said to be the father of Taoism. He described the essential nature of the 'Tao' (pronounced *Dao*), which can be loosely (but never accurately, since rather confusingly 'it can never be described') described as the abstract force responsible for creation, change and development of all things in nature, and this was recorded in the Tao Te King (pronounced *Dao De Jing*) (circa 200–100 BC). This philosophy gave rise to such modern phrases as 'go with the flow' and 'the journey of a thousand miles begins with one step'. The idea is to very much go where nature takes you or 'flow like the river, be still like the mountain'. The Chinese believed in the concept of the Tao rather than any form of deity.

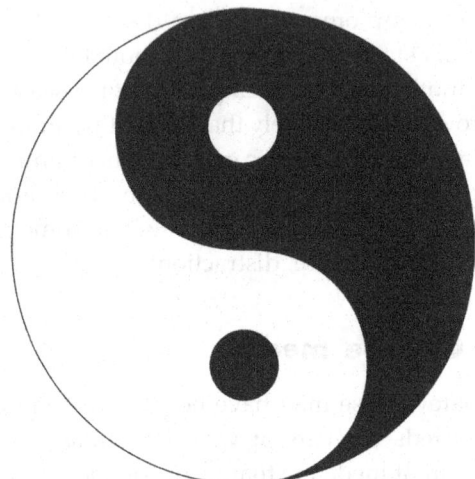

Figure 2.1 Yin and Yang symbol.

The concept of Yin & Yang was derived from a lesser-known philosophy called Naturalism, rather than from Taoism, but the Chinese of the time favoured syncretism rather than sectarianism, so new ideas were incorporated into the existing system. Yin & Yang is the fundamental duality that is thought to exist throughout the natural world. The Tao brings out the polarity between Yin & Yang from an unstructured primal state. Yin & Yang are opposites that complement each other in a dynamic process and this familiar symbol is shown in Figure 2.1. The original meaning of Yang is reflected in the old Chinese ideogram: it is the sunny (fertile) side of the hill, while Yin symbolises the shady side.

Qi (pronounced *chi*) is the life energy or vital force. It is omnipresent in nature and is apparent in all things in the form of life and movement. It is both innate (inherited) and acquired from food and respiration. It accumulates in the organs and flows around the body in channels or meridians. Qi is said to flow along meridians in a specific pattern, regulating bodily functions and nourishing the organs. It is thought that disease occurs when the flow of Qi is disturbed by certain pathologies, which include damp, cold, wind and phlegm. By needling points along the meridians it is possible to influence the flow of Qi, and thus exert a therapeutic effect on the body. There are 12 paired meridians (i.e. on each side of the body) and two

unpaired ones (in the midline), making 14 in total. It is also important to note that the needling of points and balancing of Qi energy
worked to maintain health. Patients were not therefore always, strictly
speaking, patients (patient means 'one who suffers') but people
seeking to avoid illness by keeping their bodies in a state of harmo-
nious balance.

In addition to the concept of duality defined by Yin & Yang,
the system of Five Phases (originally mistakenly translated as 'Five
Elements') was introduced. While Yin & Yang is useful in understanding polar processes, the Five Phases allows categorisation of
processes that display a phasic course. These Phases are wood, fire,
earth, metal and water. They are intimately linked in that each stimulates the next phase in the cycle, but controls or inhibits the following one. This system is thought to have originated in India, and
spread to China with the flowering of Buddhism [circa 100–
600 AD].

Pulse and tongue diagnosis was probably developed under the
influence of Confucianism, which held that the body was sacred and
therefore not to be exposed. Physicians of the time were probably
required to make an assessment of their patient by careful examination of the exposed parts of the head, lower arms and lower legs. This
may also help to explain why there are so many hand and foot points
deemed to be of importance in TCM, when many Western practitioners use these less frequently.

In TCM theory, cold and damp are thought to sometimes cause
disease; it is thought, therefore, that heat can help to banish these
pathologies from the body. Heating of points is achieved by burning
a herb: *Artemesia vulgaris* or 'moxa'. Moxa burns slowly and has a
distinctive smell. This technique is called moxibustion. Moxa can be
burnt in a roll and held near to a point, or burnt on a slice of ginger
placed on the required point. Sometimes it is burnt on the end of a
needle. In the East, a technique termed 'cauterising moxibustion' is
still often used. This involves burning a small quantity of the herb
placed in direct contact with the patient's skin, with the specific intent
of causing a burn.

Moxibustion is used in the West, but in the context of orthodox
medical practice the technique has three major drawbacks: it has been
associated with burns, the smell is not only distinctive, but rather suggestive of illicit substances, and the smoke tends to trigger fire alarms.
In veterinary practice, the additional potential for setting fire to
animal fur means that moxibustion will not be described beyond this
paragraph.

The use of traditional Chinese medicine in veterinary practice

Until recently, it was impossible to formally learn veterinary acupuncture without being exposed to elements of TCM, or TCM in its entirety. It is therefore unsurprising that a large number of veterinary practitioners use aspects of TCM in their acupuncture practice. Some practitioners embrace all elements of TCM in their practice, while others use selected ideas, for example: some schools emphasise the Five Phases over other aspects of TCM. Commonly, in the West, an orthodox diagnosis is reached and TCM principles applied: a so-called 'combined approach'.

There is much argument, discussion and controversy about elements of TCM. Certain factions place a good deal of emphasis on the principles of 'energetics'; others dismiss this as a more recent phenomenon based on the mistranslation of Chinese texts. Some of those who have translated the texts claim that all along the Chinese were describing vessels, nerves and tendons, and it is the original translators who have substituted channels and meridians, thereby creating years of misunderstanding.

What can be said with confidence is that TCM is an empirical system based on observation of clinical phenomena, response and examination. It includes a system of diagnosis or assessment, and therapy is constructed on an individual basis. Since the diagnoses are not based on Western premise, an unlimited number of conditions can be treated. Death is natural and the emphasis is on maintaining health rather than treating disease. Because of this and because all elements, including psychosocial factors, are taken into account, the approach is seen as more 'holistic' than that taken by Western medicine, be it veterinary or human. Whether this is really the case, and the actual definition of holism, is the subject of a much wider argument.

ACUPUNCTURE COMES TO THE WEST

In the years of the latter part of the seventeenth century, the Dutch East India company employed a young doctor by name of Wilhelm Ten Rhyne. In those days it was difficult to persuade physicians to accompany sea voyages; sea travel was arduous, dangerous and disease was rife. It therefore became advantageous to offer physicians some hold space on board ship so that they could purchase silks, spices and other goods with which they could greatly enhance their wealth and balance the bodily risks against the potential for material gain.

While in the Dutch trading post on Deshima at Nagasaki, Ten Rhyne observed acupuncture and was both intrigued and impressed. On his return to England he wrote his treatise *Dissertatio de Arthritide: Mantissa Schematica: De Acupunctura: . . .*[3], which, while it was not the first work to mention acupuncture in the West, it was the first to describe it in detail. The response to this work and other publications of the time was complex and, in part, due to a misinterpretation of some of Ten Rhyne's translations. Interestingly, one of these mistranslations indicated that the needle should be placed close to the point of pain. From a Western perspective this describes local needling, but it is not at all what the Japanese text meant to convey. In the West, during the following few decades, the technique was neither dismissed nor embraced wholeheartedly. It was seen partly as an opportunity to compete with lucrative 'medical' practices, partly as a surgical technique and, due to another mistranslation of Ten Rhyne's, a form of Asian bloodletting[4].

Acupuncture probably never completely disappeared from the medical scene and achieved partial assimilation into orthodox medical practice in the nineteenth and twentieth centuries. In 1835 *The Dublin Journal* quotes an 'advance' made by one Dr Stokes. This account of galvanism and acupuncture, which technique 'at least possesses the merit of novelty', describes passing a galvanic current through acupuncture needles. What is more interesting about the description is that it is airily stated that: '. . . acupuncture is widely used and its efficacy generally accepted'[5]. This attitude is echoed in a statement by Sir William Osler in his textbook: *The Principles and Practice of Medicine*, 1892[6]. In this weighty tome Osler stated that acupuncture was one of the most effective forms of treatments for lumbago and indicated his preference for the use of hatpins as needles in what must have been a fairly potent and distracting technique.

The first veterinary acupuncture paper in Europe was published by the apparently prescient forerunner to *The Veterinary Record*, when *The Veterinarian* published a report on veterinary acupuncture in 1828.

But the real enthusiasm about acupuncture in the West came with the lifting of the so-called bamboo curtain in the 1970s. After Nixon's visit to China, incredulous reports of surgery carried out on happy, smiling patients, apparently kept pain free only by acupuncture, were carried back by word and film by Western reporters and observers.

The original enthusiasm for electroacupuncture as an adjunct to, or replacement for, anaesthesia has waned with experience, but at least one reason for the popularity of the basic technique being maintained this time around (aside from enhanced communication) is undoubtedly the embracing of all things Eastern, alternative and natural by the 'stressed' and driven West, looking for other approaches to life and disease and for diversions from life in the fast lane.

ACUPUNCTURE IS INTRODUCED TO THE VETERINARY PROFESSION

In the 1970s veterinarians could only learn acupuncture by travelling to China to be taught there and a surprising number of committed individuals did just that. After the formation of the International Veterinary Acupuncture Society in 1974, courses run by the Society increasingly became available slightly closer to home, although attendance still entailed a good deal of travelling and commitment; the time required to master the breadth of information available on TCM is daunting.

MERIDIANS AND POINTS

Traditional Chinese medicine concepts describe all human body parts as being interconnected by collaterals and channels known as meridians, and the acupuncture points are found on these. There are 12 major bilaterally distributed meridians and each meridian is linked to an organ. There are eight extra meridians (also sometimes referred to as channels or vessels), which are not associated with organs, the most important of these are the Conception vessel, which runs down the centre of the front of the body and the Governing vessel, which runs up the centre of the back. An example of a human meridian is shown in Figure 2.2. Each acupuncture point has a Chinese name, which not only describes its position but also its function. However, for simplicity and for universal ease of use a numerical system has been accepted. The order of numbering is determined by the direction of flow of Qi along the channels, so that some meridians are numbered from the extremity towards the body and others numbered from the body to the extremity.

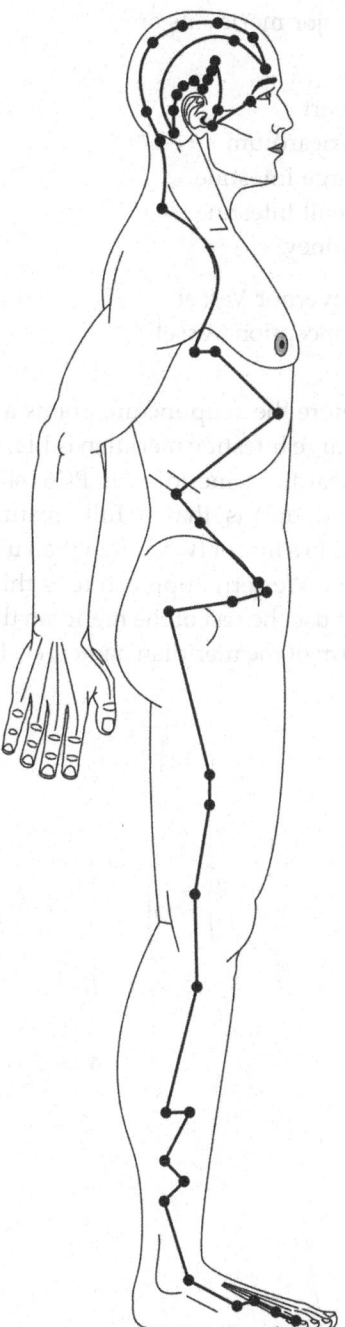

Figure 2.2 Example of a human meridian line: this shows the Gall Bladder meridian, which is said to run from the lateral aspect of the head to the foot.

The major meridians are:

LU = Lung

HT = Heart

PC = Pericardium

LI = Large Intestine

SI = Small Intestine

KI = Kidney

TE = Triple Energiser

ST = Stomach

BL = Bladder

GB = Gall Bladder

SP = Spleen

LR = Liver

GV = Governor Vessel

CV = Conception Vessel

Therefore the acupuncture points are named thus: the fourth point on the Large Intestine meridian is LI4, shown in Figure 2.3, the sixth on the Pericardium meridian is PC6, shown in Figure 2.4. This useful shorthand means that a full treatment can be communicated or recorded in a line or two, rather than using lengthy anatomical descriptions. The Western approach uses this nomenclature, even though it does not use the rest of the meridian theory and tends to use the shortened form of the meridian names, i.e. LI instead of Large Intestine.

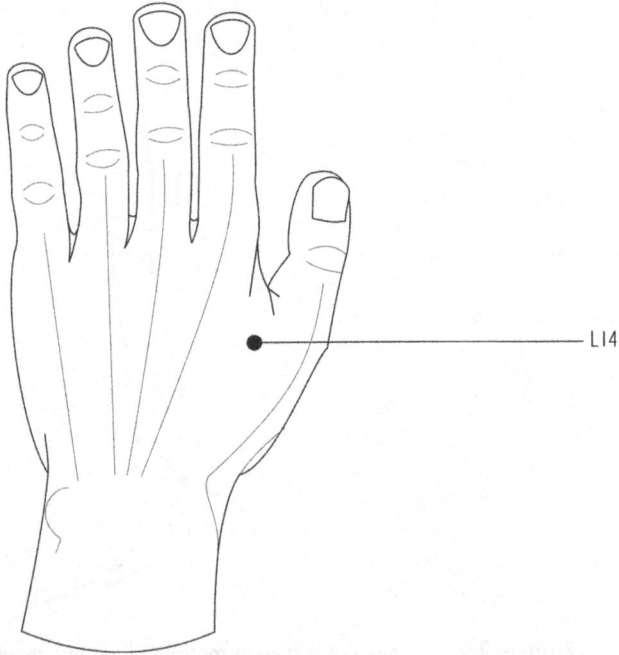

Figure 2.3 The point LI4, or Large Intestine 4, in humans is in the first dorsal interosseous muscle.

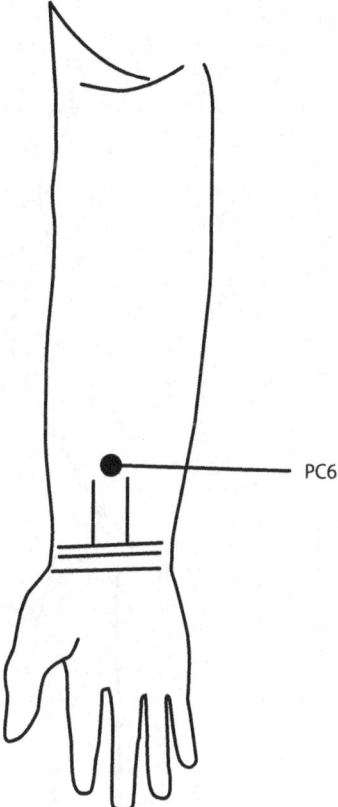

PC6

Figure 2.4 The point PC6, or Pericardium 6, in humans is located 2 cun above the distal wrist crease, between the tendons of flexor carpi radialis and palmaris longus.

For the reader of this text who has no training in traditional concepts, it is easier to think of the point names or numbers simply as ways of communicating information about where the needles are placed. The meridians often seem to bear no anatomical relationship to our concept of the organs with which they are linked: for example, the Large Intestine meridian runs up the human forearm, over the shoulder and finishes by the nose, as shown in Figure 2.5. From the Western perspective it can be difficult to conceive of organs that sound familiar by name, but not by function, or of 'organs' that are unrecognisable altogether, such as the Triple Energiser.

Meridian pathways are drawn for animals, but there is controversy about their pathways in the veterinary species. Clearly there are also

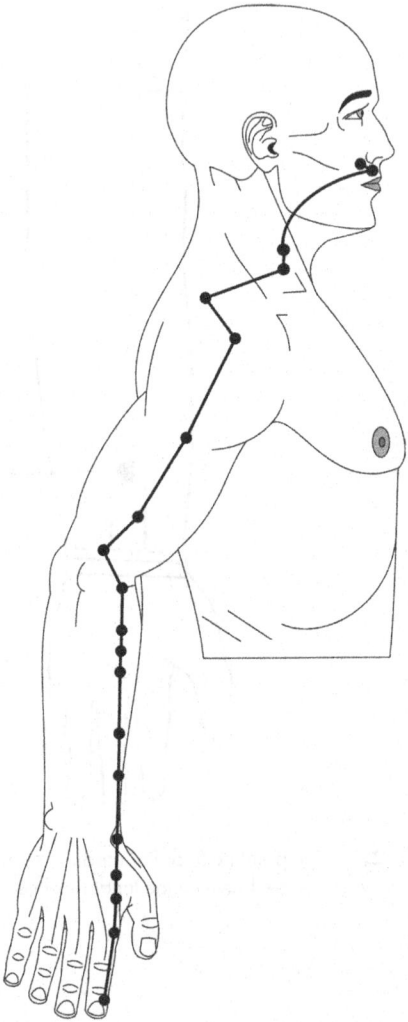

Figure 2.5 The Large Intestine meridian.

some significant anatomical discrepancies between humans and animals. For example, the popular and commonly used point LI4 is found in the first dorsal interosseous muscle of humans, and shown in Figure 2.3; this muscle is insignificant in dogs and the point is found in the small amount of soft tissue adjacent to the dew claw, or where the dew claw might have been, shown in Figure 2.6. In horses, there is no muscle at this point at all (Figure 2.7). From the Western perspective one must question the neurophysiological significance of

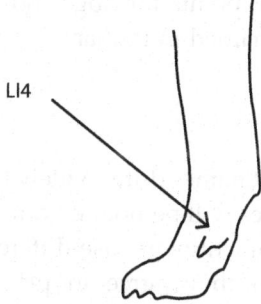

Figure 2.6 LI4 in dogs is located between the dew claw and the second metacarpal bone.

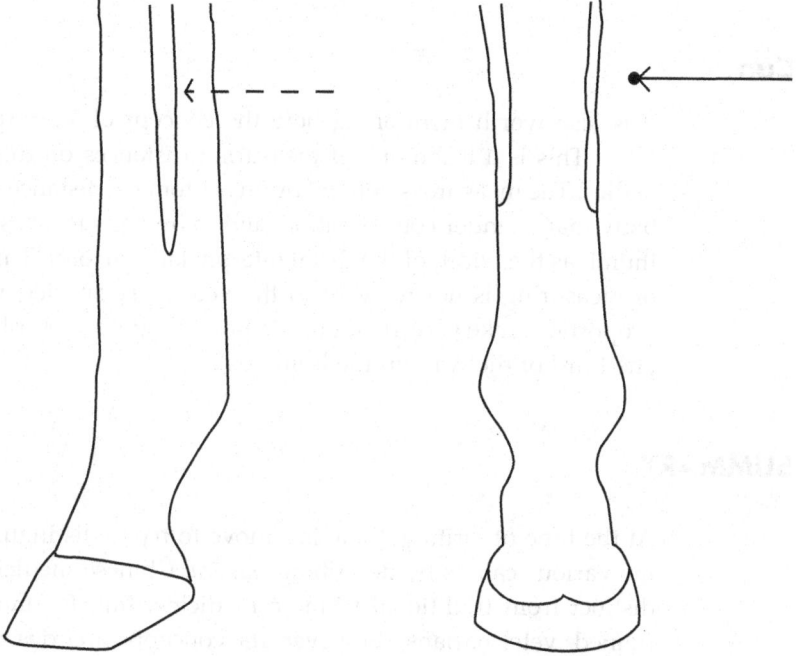

Figure 2.7 LI4 in the horse: the broken arrow on the medial view and the arrow and point on the caudal view demonstrate that the equivalent anatomical point would not technically exist in the horse since there is no first metacarpal bone or first dorsal interosseous muscle.

needling this point in these species compared with the profound sensation and potential psychological effects of stimulating the first dorsal interosseous muscle in humans.

In any case, where charts do describe points for animals the numbers are significantly smaller than in man; for instance some will give only 76 points for dogs and 173 for horses, compared with the 366 points named in humans.

Point positions

Where point names differ widely from those given in other texts these discrepancies will be pointed out. In any case it is clear that, in practice, most practitioners use different sites for points whose anatomical position they agree in principle. From a neurophysiological viewpoint every animal is 'wired up' slightly differently and some disease processes (e.g. osteoarthritis) will distort the anatomy, so insistence on precise and reproducible points to within millimetres of each other seems unnecessarily dogmatic.

Cun

It is also worth mentioning here the concept of 'cun' (pronounced *tsun*). This is a technique of measuring distances on different sized bodies. The measure is defined by an anatomical distance on the same body that is under consideration, and in humans is measured on the thumb as the width of the distal interphalangeal joint. This technique of measuring is not relevant in the veterinary species, where body proportions take precedence (e.g. a point might be described as being one-third of the way up the humerus).

SUMMARY

At the time of writing, there is a move to try to distinguish between the various camps by describing *classical* Chinese medicine as being distinct from traditional Chinese medicine. But, for most Western-trained veterinarians, however its concepts are described, TCM requires a paradigm shift in thinking, if not a leap of faith. In the opinion of the authors of this book, such a leap is not necessary. For those who enjoy mystery, there are mysteries aplenty in the mammalian nervous system and these probably have more chance of being unravelled. We would argue that it is valid to approach acupuncture from a purely neurophysiological viewpoint and still have success in treating clinical problems.

It may be true to say (though this has not been verified objectively) that those using a TCM approach get better results overall, but this would not be surprising since there are more *non-specific effects* of such treatment. It is also likely that other issues are addressed during TCM consultations, such as diet, which may have a significant impact on disease or signs of disease.

Essentially there can only be so many pathways that are activated by afferent stimuli (and acupuncture is an afferent (incoming) stimulus). Eastern, Western, or 'combined approach' practitioners, with or without a belief in Energetics, tend to stick their needles in the same places in the body and achieve broadly the same results (when depth, stimulation and condition are accounted for).

It is the opinion of the authors that if acupuncture is a useful tool that can benefit patients then it should be accessible. If taking a neurophysiological approach achieves positive results then it is valid to take this approach. If such an approach convinces more veterinarians to learn acupuncture or to refer patients for acupuncture then these are valid reasons for its adoption.

Since many TCM practitioners claim that their individual approach is not conducive to inclusion in Western research programmes, then encouraging a neurophysiological approach should yield better research and help us to achieve more quickly the answer to that ever sticky question – *does acupuncture work*?

REFERENCES

1. Dorfer L, Moser M, Spindler K, Bahr F, Egarter-Vigl E, Dohr G. 5200-year-old acupuncture in central Europe? *Science* 1998;282(5387):242–3.
2. Dorfer L, Moser M, Bahr F, Spindler K, Egarter-Vigl E, Giullen S, Dohr G, Kenner T. A medical report from the stone age? *Lancet* 1999;354(9183):1023–5.
3. Ten Rhyne W. *Dissertatio de Arthritide: Mantissa Schematica: De Acupunctura.* London: Royal Society; 1683.
4. Bivins R. *Acupuncture, Expertise and Cross-Cultural Medicine.* Basingstoke: Palgrave; 2000.
5. Hamilton J. Account of a trial of acupuncture with galvanism, made by Dr W Stokes, a physician to the Meath Hospital. *The Dublin Journal* 1835.
6. Osler W. *The Principles and Practice of Medicine.* New York: D Appleton; 1892.

Acupuncture – what is it and how does it work?

DEFINITION OF ACUPUNCTURE

The term acupuncture is derived from its Latin roots: *acus* for needle and *punctura* for penetrate. Therefore, by definition, anything that involves neither a needle nor penetration of the skin is not acupuncture. Terms such as non-needle acupuncture or laser acupuncture are thus misnomers, although widely used. But acupuncture is defined in different ways. The definition for the purposes of this book has already been outlined and agreed by the Acupuncture Regulation Working Group (ARWG):

> *Insertion of a solid needle into the body for the purpose of therapy, disease prevention or maintenance of health*[1].

Maintenance of health is not something that Western practitioners would usually include in their definition of acupuncture since most animals are presented with disease or pain and rarely, if ever, for prophylaxis. Indeed, many clients would look askance if such a measure were suggested by their orthodox veterinarian, and given that it has taken us years to convince many owners to maintain vaccinations, worming and health checks in the face of reasonable evidence of necessity, it would probably be a challenge too far to suggest needling as a form of health maintenance.

But other definitions of acupuncture include the interaction between therapist and patient. For the veterinary species this would also include the interaction between therapist, owner and animal. Such an interaction may affect the attitude of the owner towards their pet. This attitude may positively affect the demeanour and apparent or real response of the animal to therapy. The owner's beliefs and expectations about the therapy, not only as explained by the therapist, but by their confidence in the therapist's manner and approach, will also influence the response. These non-specific effects are important and useful, but also confound our attempts to answer the questions: what is acupuncture and does it work?

Briefly: the specific effects of acupuncture needling are mediated through **stimulation of the peripheral nervous system** and **neuro-modulation within the central nervous system** that occurs as a consequence.

NEUROPHYSIOLOGY OF PAIN

It is easier to explain acupuncture first in relation to its effects on pain. That is mainly because this is the area that we understand the best, although far from completely. Pain is defined, by the International Association for the Study of Pain[2], as:

> ... an unpleasant sensory and emotional experience, associated with actual or potential tissue damage.

The different aspects of pain will be discussed later. Here it is sufficient to review pain as a stimulus and acupuncture as another stimulus that competes with it.

Acute pain is mediated by fast, myelinated fibres. In the skin these are generally called A delta fibres; in muscle they are categorised as type II and III fibres. The purpose of these fast fibres is to signal potential or actual tissue damage. In this way the brain can recognise that damage is about to be done (for example, when one touches something hot) and react so as to limit that damage (snatch the hand away). The fast pain fibres synapse once in the dorsal horn before travelling to the brain via spinothalamic tracts. Their high-speed (12–30 m/s) transmission creates a column of positive 'contrast', stronger than transmissions from other peripheral inputs, and therefore, effectively, their 'message' gets priority. It is important to note that the pain experienced when A delta fibres are stimulated is not *aversively* painful, i.e. it does not cause feelings of depression or nausea or any of the other unpleasant emotions that are commonly associated with pain. When these fibres are stimulated in muscle, however, they are associated with feelings of heaviness, aching and sometimes numbness.

It is the slower C fibres, with their multisynaptic connections and input to the limbic system, and whose transmission follows on from that of the A delta fibres, which trigger feelings of aversion, depression and nausea. The purpose of these feelings is to induce withdrawal and rest, but also to teach the organism not to experience that sensation again, thus optimising the likelihood of survival. The A delta fibres signal potential injury and therefore optimise the likelihood that limiting action can be taken before actual tissue damage is done. The dual signalling system therefore limits damage, optimises recovery and teaches the individual to be wary of repeating the experience. A schematic view of this is shown in Figure 3.1.

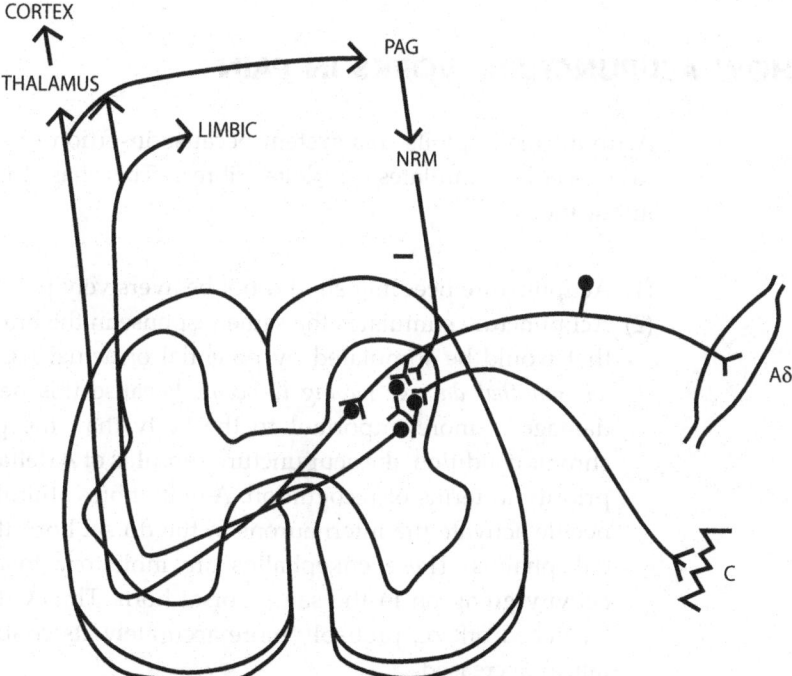

Figure 3.1 Schematic of pain transmission at the dorsal horn. Stimulation of A delta, or fast pain, fibres synapses once in the dorsal horn and continues up the crossed spinothalmic tracts, indicating potential tissue damage. Slower C fibre transmission is multisynaptic and involves the limbic system thus giving an emotional component to pain. Pain stimulates the release of endorphins from the periaqueducatal grey (PAG) and serotonin from the nucleus raphae magnus (NRM). Fibres from the NRM supply the dorsolateral funiculus to every segment of the spinal cord. This represents one of the four descending inhibitory control pathways.

Summary

(1) The recognition of acute pain is vital for survival.

(2) A delta (type III in muscle) fibres signal potential tissue damage.

(3) A delta fibre stimulation does not cause aversive pain.

(4) The aching, distension and heavy feeling that accompanies the stimulation of type III fibres in muscles equates to the so-called *de qi*, or needling sensation, which, in TCM, is said to signal a connection with the Qi and indicate that the right 'point' has been needled.

(5) C fibre stimulation causes soreness and aversive feelings, i.e. it creates the affective component of pain that makes humans and animals suffer.

HOW ACUPUNCTURE WORKS IN PAIN

Acupuncture exploits this system because insertion of an acupuncture needle stimulates A delta fibres. This has the following implications:

(1) Acupuncture needling should not be aversively painful.

(2) Acupuncture stimulates the same response in the brain and body that would be stimulated by potential or actual tissue damage, *without that damage having to occur*. Because this new potential damage is more important to the body than the pain from a chronic condition, the acupuncture stimulus of A delta fibres takes priority in terms of recognition. A delta fibres stimulated by the needle activate the interneurons in the dorsal horn that produce enkephalins. These enkephalins are inhibitory to any C fibre activity going on in the same dorsal horn. Thus C fibre pain is 'switched off' or, probably more accurately, its contrast (importance) decreased.

This event occurs in the dorsal horn of the spinal segment that has been needled. Thus getting the needle *as close as possible* to the area from which the C fibre (chronic pain) is arising should have the maximum effect by competing at the dorsal horn. This is called **segmental acupuncture** and is shown in Figure 3.2.

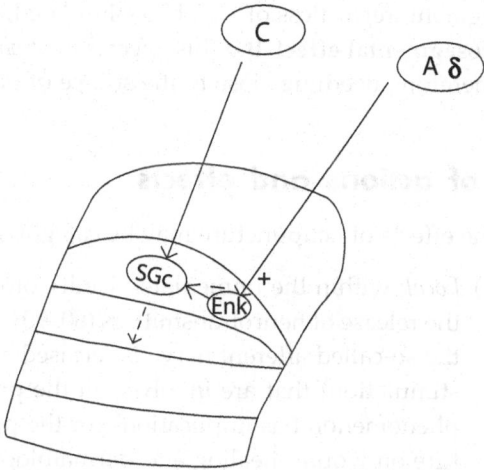

Figure 3.2 Section of the dorsal horn. Stimulation of A delta fibres results in inhibition of substantia gelatinosa cells (SGc) by enkephalinergic interneurons, thus 'closing the spinal gate' to the input of C fibres.

Effects beyond the dorsal horn

After synapsing in the dorsal horn, A delta transmission continues up the crossed spinothalamic tracts to the brain. Various interactions at this level stimulate release of the following neurotransmitters[3]:

- β endorphin from the periaqueductal grey (PAG).
- Noradrenaline indirectly from the gigantocellular reticular region (possibly locus ceruleus).
- Serotonin from the nucleus raphe magnus of the medulla oblongata.
- Oxytocin (vagal nuclei), adrenocorticotrophic hormone (ACTH) from the pituitary.

Some of these neurotransmitters act humerally, some via descending inhibitory control systems. These systems (four descending inhibitory control systems are recognised, three of them are reasonably well understood) 'damp down' the perception of pain at every spinal segment by inhibiting the transmission of painful stimuli via various mechanisms. Serotonin and noradrenaline are involved with and potentiate the effects of descending inhibitory control and therefore increase the inhibition of pain. Acupuncture results in increased activity in the descending inhibitory control systems because it is acting like a potentially damaging stimulus. This effect occurs at each spinal segment, regardless of which is stimulated, and is known as the **heterosegmental effect**. But this effect is *most potent at the segment needled*. Therefore, needling close to the source of pain is most effective.

Summary of actions and effects

The effects of acupuncture may be categorised by their site of action:

(1) *Local:* within the immediate vicinity of the needle. These include the release of neurotransmitters (80–90% of neurotransmitter from the so-called afferent nerve is released at the peripheral end after stimulation) that are involved in the promotion of healing. This phenomenon has implications for the possible effect of acupuncture on wound healing and dermatological conditions.
(2) *Segmental:* within the segment of the spinal cord where the nerves from the needled site enter the central nervous system, as described above.
(3) *Heterosegmental:* at all segmental levels of the central nervous system, as described above.
(4) *General:* this describes the effects that appear to impinge on the whole body, possibly through release of neuropeptides or hormones into the circulation (cerebrospinal fluid and vascular system).

Or effects may be categorised by the nature of their action:

Analgesic

This includes the segmental and heterosegmental effects described above, but also the deactivation of myofascial trigger points (see: Part Two). This may be through a spinal reflex mechanism similar to that which mediates the local twitch response, or it may simply be an example of segmental pain modulation.

Non-analgesic

These effects include:

(1) *Wound healing,* for which there is a relatively good evidence, both clinical and experimental[4,5] (see: Chapter 9).
(2) *Antiemesis,* for which there is evidence in humans, particularly in postoperative and post-chemotherapeutic nausea and vomiting[6,7].

(3) *Stroke rehabilitation*, around which there was considerable interest, but which has since been shown to be a non-specific effect. In other words, acupuncture provides an enriched sensory environment and it is this that speeds recovery from stroke, but any enriched environment appears to have the same effect[8,9].

(4) *Autonomic modulation*: there is evidence that acupuncture can influence the autonomic nervous system. For example: in detrusor muscle instability in man, acupuncture was shown to be as effective as the standard treatment, oxybutynin[10].

(5) *Treatment of addictions*: one of the popular images of acupuncture is that it can 'cure' all sorts of addictions, from smoking to heroin addiction. The weight of evidence is that acupuncture may have a helpful effect if the patient is suffering from withdrawal symptoms that make it difficult for them to resist the addiction, but not on the psychosocial influences that may make them return to their addiction[11,12].

(6) *Immunomodulation*: there is some evidence that acupuncture can have effects on the immune system. These effects may be similar to the positive effects of regular exercise and mediated via endorphins[13].

THE EVIDENCE FOR ACUPUNCTURE ANALGESIA

To date, we have the most information on the mechanism of acupuncture analgesia (AA). The following are a selection of the 17 lines of evidence for acupuncture analgesia recorded by Pomeranz[14]:

(1) AA requires stimulation of an intact nervous system.

(2) AA is blocked by local anaesthesia of the tissue being stimulated.

(3) AA is blocked by nerve section or nerve damage.
These three emphasise the need for an intact and functioning nervous system for acupuncture analgesia to work.

(5) AA is blocked by naloxone.

(6) AA is blocked by antibodies to endorphins.

(7) AA is blocked by microinjection of naloxone or antibodies.

(8) AA is blocked by six opiate antagonists.
These demonstrate that acupuncture analgesia works, at least partly, via the release of endogenous endorphins.

(9) AA is not affected by dextro-naloxone.
Dextro-naloxone is an optical isomer of the naturally occurring levo (left handed) form of naloxone. Dextro forms of isomers

cannot fit into the receptor sites of their natural counterparts, therefore the implication of this evidence is that endorphins are working at receptor sites.

(10) AA is subject to cross circulation effects.

Subjects connected to each other via CSF and blood both show changes when only one subject is needled.

(11) AA is associated with a rise in messenger RNA for pre-proenkephalin.

After subsequent 'doses' of acupuncture the central nervous system produces more endorphins and this can damp down the effects of central sensitisation. This is probably one of the explanations for why acupuncture appears to continue 'working' after the needles have been removed and in the presence of continuing pathology.

(12) AA is blocked by lesioning of the periaqueductal grey (PAG).

(13) AA is blocked by lesioning the arcuate nucleus.

Acupuncture works in part by the release of substances from these centres (descending inhibitory control effects).

The caveat

While all this evidence sounds very impressive, it should be pointed out that it was established for *acute* analgesia under experimental conditions on laboratory animals. The analgesic effects of acupuncture were tested against measures such as tail flick latency, during which the tail of a laboratory rat is exposed to a hot stimulus and the time taken for it to flick its tail away measured.

So, while it is probable that all the mechanisms described here *are* involved in the analgesic effects of acupuncture when treating chronic pain, it should be remembered that there is a vast difference between the short-term effects of trying to compete with the heating of a rat's tail and the clinical picture of chronic pain and suffering that occurs in, for example, a dog with chronic osteoarthritis.

THE EVIDENCE FOR ACUPUNCTURE POINTS

Traditional Chinese medicine describes very specific anatomical sites for acupuncture points and they have often been described as though they are specific entities that can be removed and scrutinised under a microscope. On the one hand, belief in this notion that 'acupoints' exist has been one of the major stumbling blocks for acupuncture research. On the other hand, the failure to cut out acupuncture points and demonstrate them histologically has been used as 'evidence' that acupuncture is so much hocus-pocus and cannot possibly work.

Some researchers are still looking for their Holy Grail of the identifiable, consistent feature that marks an acupuncture point and makes it unique, but it seems unlikely that this will ever be discovered.

Examination of the anatomical sites at which acupuncture points have been described reveals inconsistent features. However, there does appear to be a pattern in terms of 'access' to the peripheral nervous system. In other words, needling at these sites may make it more likely that a more potent stimulus is received. The more potent the stimulus, the more likely it is that it will be able to compete with the pain that is being treated at the relevant dorsal horn. Some acupuncture points are closely correlated with:

- Nerve bundles
- Nerves emerging through deep fascia
- Perivascular plexuses of nervi vasorum
- Motor points of muscle
- Myofascial trigger points
- Nerves in ligaments and joint capsules[15].

Myofascial trigger points are described in detail later, but otherwise it can be seen that all of these structures would produce a stronger stimulus when directly needled than an adjacent section of skin, muscle and fascia with none of these features. These points were probably originally described and ascribed actions because of the strong sensations produced in the patients when they were needled at these sites. If such points were also adjacent to some easily identifiable bony structure, or in a natural hollow or dip between tissues then so much the better: this made it easier to pass on the knowledge to fellow therapists.

SUMMARY

(1) Acupuncture works in painful conditions by 'fooling' the brain into thinking that potential tissue damage has just occurred.
(2) The most potent analgesic effects of acupuncture occur at the dorsal horn of the spinal segment that has been needled.
(3) For this reason, wherever possible the needle should be inserted as close as possible to the source of pain.

(4) There is evidence that acupuncture can affect wound healing, immunomodulation, emesis and autonomic function and, to a lesser extent, help with addictions.

SUMMARY OF EFFECTS

(1) Local effects
  - Afferent nerve stimulation
  - Vasodilation
  - Blood vessel proliferation
  - Nerve growth

(2) Segmental effects
  - Pain modulation
  - Autonomic modulation

(3) Heterosegmental effects
  - Enhanced descending inhibition

(4) General effects
  - Endorphin release
  - ACTH release
  - Oxytocin release

REFERENCES

1. Acupuncture Regulatory Working Group. *The Statutory Regulation of the Acupuncture Profession – The Report of the Acupuncture Regulatory Working Group.* The Prince of Wales's Foundation for Integrated Health; 2003. ISBN 0953945375.
2. Pain terms: a current list with definitions and notes on usage. In: Merskey H, Bogduk N, editors. *Classification of Chronic Pain: Descriptions of Chronic Pain Syndromes and Definitions of Pain Terms*, 2nd edn. Seattle: IASP Press; 1994. pp. 209–14.
3. Bowsher D. Mechanisms of acupuncture. In: Filshie J, White A, editors. *Medical Acupuncture: A Western Scientific Approach.* Edinburgh: Churchill Livingstone; 1998. pp. 69–82.
4. Jansen G, Lundeberg T, Samuelson UE, Thomas M. Increased survival of ischaemic musculocutaneous flaps in rats after acupuncture. *Acta Physiol Scand* 1989;135(4):555–8.
5. Lundeberg T, Kjartansson J, Samuelsson U. Effect of electrical nerve stimulation on healing of ischaemic skin flaps. *Lancet* 1988;2(8613):712–4.

6. Lee A, Done ML. The use of nonpharmacologic techniques to prevent postoperative nausea and vomiting: a meta-analysis. *Anesth Analg* 1999; 88(6):1362–9.

7. Vickers AJ. Can acupuncture have specific effects on health? A systematic review of acupuncture antiemesis trials. *J R Soc Med* 1996;89(6): 303–11.

8. Johansson BB, Haker E, von Arbin M, Britton M, Langstrom G, Terent A, Ursing D, Asplund K. Acupuncture and transcutaneous nerve stimulation in stroke rehabilitation: a randomized, controlled trial. *Stroke* 2001;32(3):707–13.

9. Park J, Hopwood V, White AR, Ernst E. Effectiveness of acupuncture for stroke: a systematic review. *J Neurol* 2001;248(7):558–63.

10. Kelleher CJ, Filshie J, Burton G, Khullar V, Cardozo ID. Acupuncture and the treatment of irritative bladder symptoms. *Acupunct Med* 1994; 12(1):9–12.

11. Marcus P. Acupuncture for the withdrawl of habituating substances. In: Filshie J, White A, editors. *Medical Acupuncture: A Western Scientific Approach*. Edinburgh: Churchill Livingstone; 1998. pp. 361–74.

12. White AR, Rampes H, Ernst E. Acupuncture for smoking cessation. *Cochrane Database Syst Rev* 2000;2:CD000009.

13. Filshie J, White A. The clinical use of, and evidence for, acupuncture in the medical systems. In: Filshie J, White A, editors. *Medical Acupuncture: A Western Scientific Approach*. Edinburgh: Churchill Livingstone; 1998. pp. 225–94.

14. Pomeranz B. Acupuncture analgesia – Neurophysiological mechanisms. *Sensory Stimulation in Pain and Diseases – International Congress at the Nobel Forum, Karolinska Institute, Stockholm, Sweden* 1997; p. 7.

15. Dung HC. Anatomic features contributing to the features of acupuncture points. *Am J Acupunct* 1984;12:139–43.

Acuncture – does it work? 4

AN EVIDENCE-BASED APPROACH

Introduction

The acceptance of acupuncture therapy into the veterinary profession will be facilitated if research is approached using the principles of evidence-based medicine (EBM). Studies must not only be scientifically rigorous, but the right questions must be asked and the results interpreted meaningfully. Methodology should address blinding, control, randomisation and outcome measures. Aside from the study protocol, other challenges include funding, ethical considerations, compliance from owners and the involvement of colleagues not *au fait* with acupuncture principles and practice.

The effectiveness pyramid

The effectiveness pyramid in Figure 4.1 illustrates what is being attempted during tests of effectiveness for any given intervention, where B represents the intervention. For our purposes B represents acupuncture. At first glance it seems logical to assume that if one starts with a symptomatic patient and applies B, then if the patient becomes asymptomatic B must be an effective intervention.

However, the picture is of course more complicated and we understand that in fact it looks like Figure 4.2, where B represents the specific effects of the treatment and the rest of the pyramid represents all the non-specific effects. For our purposes B would represent the effects of insertion of a solid needle through the skin with the inten-

45

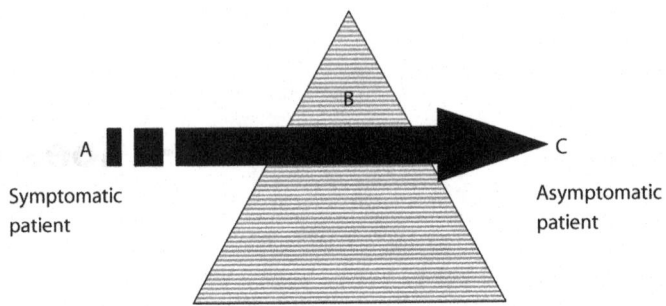

Figure 4.1 The effectiveness pyramid. B = acupuncture.

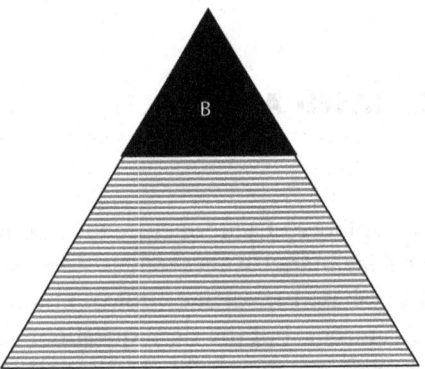

Figure 4.2 The effectiveness pyramid. B = specific effects of acupuncture.

tion of having a therapeutic effect on the signs or symptoms of A and the rest of the pyramid would include those effects that could be generated in ways not necessarily specific to acupuncture treatment.

Non-specific effects include:

Expectation (placebo)

Placebo means literally 'pleasing the patient'. While one may argue that most of our veterinary patients are far from pleased at the prospect of any veterinary intervention, animal placebo effects are accepted and must be accounted for in any trial. Although the term is often used pejoratively ('it's just placebo') placebo is a powerful neurophysiological effect, mediated in part by endorphins and can be both specifically targeted and specifically blocked. One of the important reasons for demonstrating that acupuncture has effects over and above the placebo effect is that the use of placebo treatment is assumed to be, and ought to be, completely safe. If the same effects can be achieved by not penetrating the skin by a needle (the point at which the treatment stops being safe), then acupuncture should be avoided and other ways of achieving the results explored.

In addition to the fact that just being nice to our patients may have effects on their health and the way they feel, their owners are also affected by the way in which their pets respond to the treatment and to the therapist. Many pets either become quite relaxed during acupuncture treatment or at least show remarkable enthusiasm on returning to the clinic even if they appear ambivalent about the needling itself. This is almost bound to produce positive feelings in the owner who may well feel, rightly or wrongly, that their pet is 'definitely' responding to the treatment. This has been dubbed the 'owner placebo effect' and, while not semantically correct, probably provides the correct impression.

Therapeutic relationship

There are effects other than expectation of recovery or placebo. The therapeutic relationship between patient and therapist is important in developing confidence in the technique, in the diagnosis and the prognosis. Simply believing that someone understands and cares is important in the way that human patients perceive their suffering and cope with it. It is more difficult to demonstrate the effects of this between pet and veterinarian since few pets would voluntarily make their way to the clinic. However, it is not inconceivable that the interaction between veterinarian and patient, especially in terms of touch and examination, could have a positive effect. Touch appears to be a potent intervention: it has been demonstrated that the release of oxytocin is triggered by light stroking to the ventral surface of rats[1]. Oxytocin is associated not only with bonding, but also with sedation, anxiolysis and analgesia. Other neurotransmitters, specifically noradrenaline, endorphins and dopamine are also released during interactions between humans and dogs[2]. While it is not possible to say with confidence whether these chemicals are the *cause* of the apparent mutual pleasure of a human–animal interaction, it seems likely that they have some part to play. Since reduction in blood pressure and increase in mood neurotransmitters occur in both human and dog, whether that human is a stranger to the dog or not, there is at least the possibility that the veterinary interaction is an important one over and above the specific therapy chosen.

Natural history

Disease processes run a natural course. Many of them appear to either wax and wane in severity over time and season (atopy and osteoarthritis, for example) or improve to an acceptable level over time or simply resolve. The tendency is to seek help when the disease process or signs are at their most severe; it is likely that after this peak the problem will settle down for a while. If an intervention has occurred around this time then it is natural that the owner and probably the therapist will attribute the improvement to the specific therapy.

Chance

At any given time it is possible that a disease or set of signs is going to spontaneously resolve and that resolution may, on occasion, coincide with the application of a given intervention.

It is difficult not to be convinced by one's own clinical observations. The 'miracle cure' will convince the most cynical of practitioners, sometimes to a point above all reason and the cynic becomes evangelist. Neither extreme is particularly helpful when trying to realistically evaluate the specific effect of acupuncture.

Error in clinical observation

The problem with clinical observation is that it is subject to numerous possible errors and these can be classified as follows:

Bias

The Cochrane Handbook refers to four sources of systematic bias in trials of the effects of healthcare and these are briefly described below[3]. The handbook makes the following statement about bias:

> *Unfortunately, we do not have strong empirical evidence of a relationship between trial outcomes and specific criteria or sets of criteria used to assess the risk of these biases[4,5]. There is, however, a logical basis for suspecting such relationships and good reason to consider these four potential biases when assessing studies for a review[6].'*

(1) *Selection bias:* For example, choosing patients that one knows from experience are likely to 'do well' with a particular treatment.

(2) *Performance bias:* Refers to systematic differences in the care provided to the participants in the comparison groups other than the intervention under investigation.

(3) *Attrition bias:* Refers to systematic differences between the comparison groups in the loss of participants from the study.

(4) *Measurement or detection bias:* Detection bias refers to systematic differences between the comparison groups in outcome assessment.

Chance

At any given time it is possible that a disease or set of signs is going to resolve spontaneously and that resolution may, on occasion, coincide with the application of a given intervention.

Confounding

Confounding factors may include concurrent treatments and changes in the environment (for example: the owner of the atopic dog may just have removed all the carpets from the house).

Because of all these factors, and despite the fact that miracle cures will continue to convert cynics and reinforce believers, there is a generally accepted hierarchy of evidence at the bottom of which is clinical observation. Academics will not consider evidence below the level of randomised controlled trial, but this does not mean that the rest have no value. Clinical observation is what gets veterinarians/therapists/medics excited and interested, case series add a little more credence to their observations and positive outcomes to cohort and controlled trials support the need and encourage funding for further research.

Hierarchy of evidence

Systematic review

This replaces the literature review written by a noted specialist or expert on the subject. In a systematic review the authors must determine the methods (how they will search for, include or exclude, and analyse the studies they are going to examine) before they start. In theory this means that studies that do not support the view of the author cannot be overlooked. There are still disagreements and the potential for flawed interpretation, but this is considered to be the highest level of evidence.

Meta-analysis

This is a way of combining the results of more than one trial in such a way as to give more confidence in the statistical outcomes.

Randomised controlled trial

This is where assessors and subjects are blinded as to the intervention received ('real' or otherwise), where patients are allocated to each arm of the trial randomly and where there is a comparison with either no treatment or another treatment.

Controlled trial

The treatment is compared with another intervention or no treatment but the patients are not randomised to each arm of the study, therefore selection bias is a possibility.

Cohort study

This is a prospective study with no controls and no randomisation but it removes the error that is due to faulty memory in a retrospective study.

Case series

These are usually retrospective and therefore rely on the memory of the clinician in recording and remembering cases.

Clinical observation

The single case that persuades clinicians and our clients that something 'definitely works', but that is subject to all the vagaries of placebo and other non-specific effects.

However rigorous, methods don't lead to good results if the original idea is faulty.

Developing a research question

Here is a typical example of a clinical research question:

Does acupuncture work in condition X?

This sounds reasonable and seems to cover what one wants to know. But what is meant in this question (and therefore by the researcher) by acupuncture? Acupuncture has been defined as:

Insertion of a solid needle into the body for the purpose of therapy, disease prevention or maintenance of health[7].

But others may include the therapeutic relationship in their definition of acupuncture: the intention to heal on the part of the therapist and the expectation of recovery on the part of the patient (or owner). Traditional or classical Chinese medicine practitioners would include in their definition of acupuncture the application of TCM principles and the needling of specific anatomical sites (acupuncture points) before the definition would satisfy them. If a study were to conclude that, for instance, acupuncture works for osteoarthritis, the practitioner would need to know which definition of acupuncture was used in order to be able to have a chance at reproducing either the effects or the study.

Once acupuncture has been defined for the purposes of the study, so that the reader *knows what has been done*, what does the question mean by 'does it work'?

It might be assumed that by using the term 'working' it is meant that the intervention cures the condition, but the therapist may only be looking to alleviate symptoms or signs, or to ameliorate only one sign. So the outcome measures must be defined and there must be a valid way of determining these. Any scoring system should ideally be validated and at least be defined; for example, just stating 'excellent' as a result is not helpful unless we know whether excellent means a cure or a satisfactory resolution of signs or that the patient just enjoyed the treatment tremendously and recommended the therapist to all and sundry.

The other point that needs to be decided is whether the study is trying to determine efficacy of an intervention or the effectiveness of an intervention. Put simply: **efficacy** is tested against 'placebo' whereas **effectiveness** is tested against an active or inactive comparator.

Finally, from this clinical research question 'condition X' must be able to be reliably defined.

After asking the right question, which is arguably the most important aspect of clinical research, there are other challenges that need to be addressed on the way to a well conducted trial. These challenges are discussed in the next section of this chapter.

CHALLENGES OF ACUPUNCTURE RESEARCH

Methodological

Blinding

Physical therapies are difficult to blind simply because it is hard to convince a patient that they have received a physical intervention, be it a needle inserted or a manipulation, when they have not. In research on humans there have been various methods used to attempt to mimic the feeling of acupuncture when acupuncture is not actually being given. Tapping on the skin with a guide tube and pinching the skin in areas where the patient cannot see what is going on have been shown in some studies to be convincing. Since the development of the sham needle, shown in Figure 4.3, it has been possible for patients to see themselves apparently being needled, when in fact the shaft of the needle disappears into the handle in the manner of a stage dagger. The disadvantage of this needle is that it obviously cannot be left in place unless supported, which means that all needles, real or otherwise, must be introduced through a supporting device, of which there are several versions; the Park unit is shown in Figure 4.4.

Who else should be blinded? It may not be necessary to blind the acupuncturist so long as the assessors are blinded. In veterinary research it is important to note that owner attitude can affect a pet's response to any treatment so that whether or not owners are being asked to assess some aspect of the condition they should also be blinded. Owners can be blinded to the intervention used by removing their pets from them for treatment. (They must first understand that treatment will be different between groups. Recruitment for acupuncture trials may be high if everyone mistakenly assumes that their pet will receive acupuncture.) However, since they must have no idea whether their pets have received acupuncture it may be necessary to consider that owners should be acupuncture naïve. Most owners whose pets have had acupuncture (and possibly those owners who have had acupuncture themselves) will be aware that there is often a post-treatment sedation effect and in some cases this is profound. The blinding procedure will be affected if the owners recognise this response. If a blinding technique is used (e.g. placebo needles) then it should be tested, i.e. the owners should be asked whether or not they believe that their pets have received acupuncture.

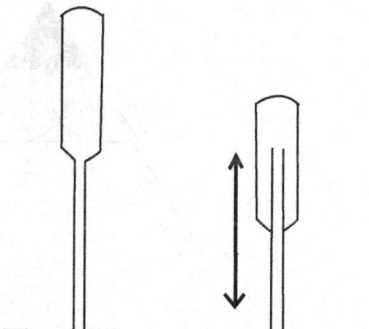

Figure 4.3 The sham or placebo needle. The needle has a blunt end and the shaft 'disappears' into its handle in the manner of a stage dagger.

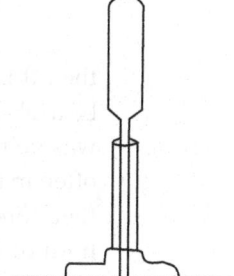

Figure 4.4 The Park sham device consists of a plastic ring and outer tube to hold the sham needle in place.

While removing pets from their owners appears to be a simple and effective method of blinding the owners to the treatment used it could be hypothesised that the anxiety felt by some animals on being separated from their owners at the clinic may interfere with the outcome of the treatment.

Controls

The control procedure should ideally mimic every aspect of the acupuncture treatment short of the needling. It should be considered whether or not the control procedure might have an effect – specific or otherwise. To date, using an active *needling* control remains the single most frequent error in acupuncture research, be it veterinary or medical. Before the advent of the 'placebo needle' the most effective way to convince patients that they were having acupuncture was to needle them. It was (and still is in some quarters) believed that if the needles were placed 'off point', or not in a classical acupuncture point,

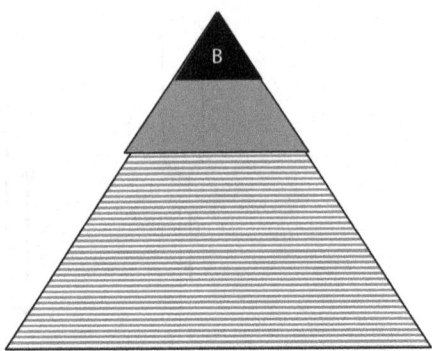

Figure 4.5 As is illustrated in here, one is trying to demonstrate B in the tiny triangle at the top of the pyramid – an effect over and above not only all the non-specific effects, but all the assumed specific neurophysiological effects of needling as well.

then this was not acupuncture and therefore could be considered to be a placebo control. In many cases this 'sham' form of acupuncture was being performed a few millimetres from the 'real' acupuncture, often in the same myotome. From the neurophysiological perspective, therefore, A delta signals from both needles would enter the dorsal horn of the same spinal segment and modulate C fibre activity in the same way. In terms of higher centres, the brain would perceive much the same stimulus and presumably respond in the same way. If both the 'sham' group and the 'real treatment' group improved with no significant difference between the two then it was concluded that acupuncture did not work . . .

By literally missing the point many studies have failed to demonstrate an effect of acupuncture that is better than that of a control assumed to be a placebo.

As is illustrated in Figure 4.5, one is trying to demonstrate B in the tiny triangle at the top of the pyramid – an effect over and above not only all the non-specific effects, but all the assumed specific neurophysiological effects of needling as well.

In other studies, where this problem has been recognised, attempts have been made to limit the effect of needling in the control subjects by using techniques such as minimal needling, i.e. very brief, superficial needling compared with needling deeply into muscle, or superficial needling compared with strong electroacupuncture. In these cases the hope is that the difference in levels of stimulation will be sufficient to show significant differences in neurophysiological effects.

Treatment approach

It should be made clear whether or not the treatment is based on assessment of an individual or whether or not a standard approach has been used. The former approach is likely to achieve better results in each case, although the latter is likely to make interpretation of the results more straightforward.

Outcome measures

Are there validated, objective ways of measuring whether the treatments have been effective?

Practical

Funding

Acupuncture is not a natural draw for funding in the veterinary profession, so most trials are small. The 'catch-22' is that funding may be available from trusts and foundations if clinical improvement in clinical conditions that cause animal suffering can be demonstrated. Funds may be available from other sources if an improvement in production or performance can be demonstrated. However, until funding is available, research is limited to small trials, the results of which may not be significant or may only indicate a trend. If those involved in research can demonstrate that acupuncture may augment other therapies or that its use means that clients stay within the influence of the profession, or are more likely to continue using, for example, a particular non-steroidal anti-inflammatory drug rather than changing between different types in the hope of an improved response, other potential sources, including even drug companies, may be prepared to look at funding.

Ethical considerations

UK veterinary schools have ethical committees looking at the potential welfare problems associated with any trial carried out within the school. A rigorous study will include a control group and in some human studies this may be the waiting list or a group given a true placebo. Animals cannot choose to take the chance of being in the non-treatment arm of a trial, so for any group in the study one must demonstrate an intention to treat. Any veterinarian thinking of conducting a study should check that they are not inadvertently straying into the situation of requiring a Home Office Licence.

Ethical considerations will usually therefore mean that a given study will be comparing one treatment (usually the standard accepted treatment) with acupuncture therapy; or compare standard treatment with standard treatment plus acupuncture. In other words such a study will be looking at *effectiveness*. This may provide useful pragmatic and clinical information, but it should be noted that it would not yield information about the *specific efficacy* of acupuncture. In other words such a study will not prove that it is the insertion of the acupuncture needle that is bringing about the change in a given clinical condition.

SUMMARY

Common pitfalls of acupuncture research

(1) The assumption that acupuncture points are specific anatomical sites.
(2) That acupuncture points unarguably have a specific effect on the body or on a clinical sign or symptom.
(3) That 'non-acupuncture points' are therefore inactive and have no specific effects on clinical problems.
(4) The consequent use of actual needling as so-called 'sham needling' in the control population without considering that this will have a real effect on the body.
(5) Failure to define or identify clinical conditions accurately.
(6) Failure to identify useful and validated outcome measures (pain scores, etc.).

In clinical trials of acupuncture

(1) Define exactly what you mean by 'acupuncture' before considering the methods.
(2) In efficacy studies: don't miss the point!

When reading and assessing research papers

Read the methods and materials section, i.e. find out what was done.

THE CURRENT STATE OF MEDICAL ACUPUNCTURE RESEARCH

This is potentially a huge subject and is outside the remit of this book on veterinary acupuncture. However there have been some significant advances in the last few years and in 2004 there was a much-publicised study published in the *British Medical Journal* demonstrating specific efficacy of acupuncture in the treatment of osteoarthritis of the human knee[8]. This has been followed by other studies, the largest at time of writing with 570 subjects, demonstrating efficacy during and at the end of weekly interventions for 26 weeks[9]. And finally, a third large randomised controlled trial was published in the *Lancet*[10].

It seems clear that acupuncture also has specific effects in the treatment of nausea and vomiting[11], particularly that occurring in the postoperative period[12]. Also, a high quality pragmatic study on acupuncture for chronic idiopathic headache demonstrates both effectiveness and cost-utility by NHS standards[13,14].

THE CURRENT STATE OF VETERINARY ACUPUNCTURE RESEARCH

One of the authors of this book (SL) is currently conducting two acupuncture-related trials at Glasgow University Veterinary School. One is an attempt to demonstrate interrater reliability in finding myofascial trigger points in dogs after the study by Gerwin *et al.*[15]. The other is a randomised, double blind, controlled trial on comparing the treatment of acral lick dermatitis by a standard approach with the standard approach plus acupuncture. Both trials demonstrate beautifully the difficulties and challenges of clinical research of any kind, but also continue to uncover previously unrecognised problems in clinical veterinary acupuncture research, some of which have been described in the earlier sections of this chapter.

As it stands there is no convincing evidence that acupuncture works for any given clinical condition in the veterinary species. Of course, much of the rigorous experimental work has been carried out on rats and rabbits, but one cannot directly equate the results of experimental pain or wound healing with the clinical picture seen by most veterinarians.

A few more recent studies demonstrate the difficulties involved in veterinary acupuncture research. While these studies have many points in their favour and reflect in some aspects a rigorous approach, they do falter at some of the common pitfalls. These are discussed below.

Example 1

Merritt *et al.* 2002[16]: Evaluation of a method to experimentally induce colic in horses and the effects of acupuncture applied at the Guan-yuan-shu (similar to BL21) acupoint.

The aims of this trial were to evaluate a method for inducing colic in horses and to test the analgesic potential of bilateral needling of one acupuncture point. The authors considered that their method of inserting a balloon into the duodenum and inflating it was an effective model for reproducing colic pain, but that the acupuncture intervention was not sufficient to treat the pain. A glance at the abstract of the paper may cause the reader to conclude that acupuncture 'does not work' for spasmodic colic.

If one were to attempt to use acupuncture to treat a spasmodic colic (and it would not be the treatment of first or sole choice, not least because of the challenge of needling a colicking animal) one would be aiming primarily to restore function and thereby alleviate pain. (Since the cause of the pain had not been addressed it could be argued that one would actually not wish for acupuncture to achieve analgesia in this case, although that was not the issue raised by this paper.) It may be possible, by stimulating the correct segmental level for the affected viscera, to normalise function, but this could not occur with this model since the cause of the pain, i.e. the inflated balloon, is still present. It should also be noted that active electroacupuncture treatment was given for 20 minutes before balloon inflation and only continued for 5 minutes after inflation. The pain of colic is an acute and potent stimulus so it is possible that this intervention was not robust enough.

The choice of point used in this experiment was sensible when based on the general observation and philosophy of traditional approaches. There is another perspective however: even given that our knowledge of segmental equine anatomy is limited, it is unlikely that stimulation of relatively superficial musculature at this point could compete at the dorsal horn of the correct spinal segment to affect pain arising from the duodenum or to modify its function.

Given these considerations, it may be unfair to decide on this basis that acupuncture does not work for colic. The authors too thought it may be an unfair conclusion: they suggested that their choice of site, use of a single point and/or choice of frequency may have not been optimal for the condition, rather than concluding that acupuncture was not a useful therapy.

Example 2

Hielm-Bjorkman *et al.* 2001[17]: Double-blind evaluation of implants of gold wire at acupuncture points in the dog as a treatment for osteoarthritis induced by hip dysplasia.

This trial looked at 38 dogs, randomly assigned to two groups of 19. The treatment group had gold wires implanted at acupuncture points roughly equivalent to GB30, BL54 and GB29 (this notation does not equate to similar points in humans), located by a point finder. The control group had the skin pierced at 'non points' around the hip with a needle the same size as that used to deliver the gold implants, i.e. 14 G. The dogs were assessed over a 6-month period by two veterinarians and the dogs' owners, none of whom knew to which group the dogs had been assigned. There were significant improvements in signs of pain and locomotion as observed by vets and owners, but no significant difference between the groups. The authors discuss a number of reasons as to why both groups improved, including the fact that the trial was conducted between March and September – warmer weather has been observed to have a positive effect on the signs of arthritis in dogs and the fact that all owners received advice regarding their dogs' weight and exercise management. They also noted that chronic conditions naturally change over time and that since both groups had interventions there could have been both an animal and owner 'placebo' response for both groups. The authors also acknowledged that the control intervention may have been active.

This was not, strictly speaking, a trial of acupuncture since the needles used were not acupuncture needles, but hypodermic 14 G needles likely to cause significant trauma to surrounding tissues. The comparison made here was of trauma to soft tissues local to the painful site versus trauma to the local site plus some inert implants. The protocol was based upon the assumption that acupuncture points are specific entities and relied on the change in skin resistance at certain sites to confirm the location of these points. From a neurophysiological perspective both interventions were likely to have a similar effect.

This trial was useful in that the results suggest that there is nothing to be gained by using gold implants in treatment, but above and beyond this it does not demonstrate whether there was a specific effect of needling, or indeed of treating the dogs at all. The main difficulty with this trial is that it would be included in any search looking for acupuncture in veterinary medicine. The abstract implies that there is no difference between a 'sham' treatment and a 'real' treatment and the conclusion could be erroneously gathered that acupuncture does not work for the treatment of osteoarthritis secondary to hip dysplasia.

SUMMARY

(1) Clinical research is challenging in any field of veterinary medicine and surgery, but there are some unique challenges with trials of acupuncture.
(2) As with all papers, one should read the materials and methods section to find out what was done, rather than take the abstract or conclusions at face value.
(3) Currently there is no rigorous evidence for or against the efficacy or the effectiveness of acupuncture in any clinical setting in the veterinary species.

REFERENCES

1. Uvnas-Moberg K, Bruzelius G, Alster P, Lundeberg T. The antinociceptive effect of non-noxious sensory stimulation is mediated partly through oxytocinergic mechanisms. *Acta Physiol Scand* 1993;149(2): 199–204.
2. Odendaal J. *Pets and Our Mental Health: The Why, the What, and the How.* New York: Vantage Press; 2002.
3. The Cochrane Collaboration. *Cochrane Handbook for Systematic Reviews of Interventions 4.2.4.* 2005. Cochrane Library (accessed on 27 July 2005).
4. Moher D, Jadad AR, Nichol G, Penman M, Tugwell P, Walsh S. Assessing the quality of randomized controlled trials: an annotated bibliography of scales and checklists. *Control Clin Trials* 1995;16(1):62–73.
5. Moher D, Jadad AR, Tugwell P. Assessing the quality of randomized controlled trials. Current issues and future directions. *Int J Technol Assess Health Care* 1996;12(2):195–208.
6. Feinstein AR. *Clinical Epidemiology: The Architecture of Clinical Research.* Philadelphia: WB Saunders; 1985.
7. Acupuncture Regulatory Working Group. *The Statutory Regulation of the Acupuncture Profession – The Report of the Acupuncture Regulatory Working Group.* The Prince of Wales's Foundation for Integrated Health; 2003. ISBN 0953945375.

8. Vas J, Mendez C, Perea-Milla E, Vega E, Panadero MD, Leon JM, Borge MA, Gaspar O, Sanchez-Rodriguez F, Aguilar I, Jurado R. Acupuncture as a complementary therapy to the pharmacological treatment of osteoarthritis of the knee: randomised controlled trial. *BMJ* 2004;329(7476):1216.

9. Berman BM, Lao L, Langenberg P, Lee WL, Gilpin AM, Hochberg MC. Effectiveness of acupuncture as adjunctive therapy in osteoarthritis of the knee: a randomised, controlled trial. *Ann Intern Med* 2004;141(12):901–10.

10. Witt C, Brinkhaus B, Jena S, Linde K, Streng A, Wagenpfeil S, Hummelsberger J, Walther HU, Melchart D, Willich SN. Acupuncture in patients with osteoarthritis of the knee: a randomised trial. *Lancet* 2005;366(9480):136–43.

11. Vickers AJ. Can acupuncture have specific effects on health? A systematic review of acupuncture antiemesis trials. *J R Soc Med* 1996;89(6):303–11.

12. Lee A, Done ML. The use of nonpharmacologic techniques to prevent postoperative nausea and vomiting: a meta-analysis. *Anesth Analg* 1999;88(6):1362–9.

13. Vickers AJ, Rees RW, Zollman CE, McCarney R, Smith CM, Ellis N, Fisher P, Van Haselen R. Acupuncture for chronic headache in primary care: large, pragmatic, randomised trial. *BMJ* 2004;328(7442):744.

14. Wonderling D, Vickers AJ, Grieve R, McCarney R. Cost effectiveness analysis of a randomised trial of acupuncture for chronic headache in primary care. *BMJ* 2004;328(7442):747.

15. Gerwin RD, Shannon S, Hong CZ, Hubbard D, Gevirtz R. Interrater reliability in myofascial trigger point examination. *Pain* 1997;69(1–2):65–73.

16. Merritt AM, Xie H, Lester GD, Burrow JA, Lorenzo-Figueras M, Mahfoud Z. Evaluation of a method to experimentally induce colic in horses and the effects of acupuncture applied at the Guan-yuan-shu (similar to BL-21) acupoint. *Am J Vet Res* 2002;63(7):1006–11.

17. Hielm-Bjorkman A, Raekallio M, Kuusela E, Saarto E, Markkola A, Tulamo RM. Double-blind evaluation of implants of gold wire at acupuncture points in the dog as a treatment for osteoarthritis induced by hip dysplasia. *Vet Rec* 2001;149(15):452–6.

Part Two

The use of acupuncture for acute and chronic pain

WHAT IS PAIN?

an unpleasant sensory and emotional experience, associated with actual or potential tissue damage or expressed in terms of such damage[1]

Therefore pain has both a **sensory** and an **affective** component; however, two other components have been identified: the **cognitive** and **motor** components. These components can be summarised as follows:

(1) *Sensory:* The recognition of a painful stimulus. This component is not aversive and does not cause suffering; it merely signals tissue damage or potential tissue damage.
(2) *Affective:* This is the part of pain that causes suffering. Pain transmission involves the limbic system and therefore an emotional aspect to the recognition of pain.
(3) *Cognitive:* This is how the pain impacts on the individual in terms of anticipation and how an individual constructs a reality around the experience, for example: a human patient may worry that someone they knew had similar pain and it led to a debilitating condition; or they may worry how it will progress, what it means and how they will cope if it gets worse.
(4) *Motor:* This involves movement away from the pain or adjustments in motor activity to limit the pain, such as not bearing weight on the affected limb or moving away from a touch that is anticipated to hurt.

How do these divisions help us in our consideration of pain in animals? Is it useful to separate the sensory from the affective components of pain since surely one inevitably follows the other? In fact some of the more recent studies of the acupuncture treatment of pain in human subjects has shown that although the sensory component may not change significantly after therapy, the pain does not bother the patients as much. In other words the suffering component of pain has been reduced. Anecdotally, it has been noticed by veterinary practitioners that owners often describe positive behavioural changes in their pets after acupuncture treatment, even though their gait or exercise tolerance may not have improved much. While it could be argued that this is just a reflection of the owner wishing to see a positive improvement, it is also possible that it demonstrates a genuine reduction in suffering.

In terms of the cognitive aspect of pain, while it is assumed that animals do not have the long-term anticipation and worry that is most noticeable in human subjects, they can certainly remember situations and contexts that previously caused pain and there is some evidence that enriching the environment of animals in pain (i.e. giving them more to do and more interest) improves their behavioural pain scores (Lundeberg, personal communication). Helping patients to pay less attention to their pain and ascribe it less importance is part of the approach to dealing with chronic and refractory pain syndromes (cognitive behaviour therapy) in humans. The Pain and Rehabilitation Clinic at Glasgow University Veterinary School uses this approach as part of the treatment of chronic pain conditions.

REVIEW OF THE NEUROPHYSIOLOGY OF PAIN[2]

Pain is classified in a number of ways: physiologic or pathologic; acute or chronic; inflammatory and neuropathic. The following summary highlights and reiterates the aspects of pain neurophysiology salient to the use of acupuncture: (see also Chapter 3)

Physiologic or nociceptive pain

This can be distinguished as the pain that occurs after any nociceptive stimulus. It has a protective function and is therefore adaptive (useful for survival):

(1) High intensity stimulus activates high threshold peripheral nociceptors.

(2) This stimulus is transmitted via A delta and C fibres.

(3) A delta fibres (or type III fibres in muscle) are fast, myelinated fibres with one synapse in the spinal cord (first order neuron to dorsal horn) projecting via second and third order neurons to the cerebral cortex. These fibres transmit so-called 'fast' pain: the initial sensation perceived when, for example, one first realises that something very hot has been touched. This is the sensory component of pain and does not cause suffering.

(4) However, the same nocioceptive stimulus also activates C fibres. These smaller unmyelinated fibres are much slower to transmit their stimulus (1–2 m/s), communicate with the limbic system and give rise to so-called 'second' or 'slow' pain. Fast and slow are, of course, relative terms and in practice A delta fibre pain is followed very rapidly by the rise in nauseating, aversive, unpleasant sensation that causes one to nurse the affected area, protect it and learn, it is supposed, not to repeat the experience. This is the affective component of pain and represents suffering.

(5) Both systems are useful: the fast pain system signals potential tissue damage and therefore may activate reflex withdrawal before actual tissue damage occurs; the slow pain triggers mechanisms associated with healing and teaches the victim not to repeat an action that will diminish its fitness and viability.

(6) Both A delta and C fibres synapse in the dorsal horn of the spinal cord, in laminae I, II and V. It is here in the dorsal horn that pain modulation primarily occurs after acupuncture stimulation.

(7) The stimulus is conveyed to supraspinal centres via spinothalamic and spinoreticular tracts.

(8) The supraspinal centres affected by a painful stimulus include those in the midbrain, cerebral cortex, thalamus and hypothalamus, reticular system and periaquedcutal grey (PAG).

Descending inhibitory pathways

These modulate pain and other sensory inputs:

(1) There are four tiers: cortical and thalamic; PAG; rostral medulla and pons; medullary and spinal cord dorsal horn.

(2) Modulation of sensory input by descending inhibitory control is mediated by serotonin, noradrenaline and endorphins, among other neurotransmitters, acting at the dorsal horn.

This model of pain is well recognised, but it does tend to over simplify pain and its transmission. It tends to give the impression that a given noxious stimulus at the periphery is faithfully signalled to the brain and clearly labelled to reflect the nature and severity of that stimulus. But, as is eloquently described by Bonica[3], this is not the case. A painful stimulus at the periphery is subject to:

> . . . a variety of mechanisms modulating transmission of information about tissue damage at virtually every synaptic relay station . . .

and there are:

> . . . dynamic interactions between neurotransmitters, their receptors . . .

as well as:

> . . . inputs from periphery, spinal cord and descending control systems . . .

In other words pain is:

> . . . a low fidelity signal reaching the thalamus determining sensory-discriminative, motivational and affective, cognitive and motor responses characteristic of pain behaviour.

Pain is a 'low fidelity' signal. This means that how an animal *feels* about a given stimulus cannot be predicted because it depends upon what else is going on in its central nervous system and in its environment. It also means that pain can be influenced and modulated at a number of levels and in a variety of ways. It may be done pharmacologically or psychologically or by competing with the painful stimulus at the level of the dorsal horn by the input of another stimulus. One way of achieving the latter is by acupuncture.

Pathologic or clinical pain

Physiologic pain is not what is being dealt with in the clinical setting. In this situation the stimulus has been either long lasting or has caused significant damage or inflammation. More than ever the simple 'transmission-of-a-message' picture of pain is distorted. There are changes to the central nervous system as the sensitivity of receptors is altered; the perception of the pain by the subject is changed and the different components of pain may actually contribute to the pain as it is experienced by the sufferer. Clinical pain is often divided into acute and chronic pain.

(1) *Acute pain:* An example of this is post-surgical pain. This facilitates tissue repair and healing by hypersensitising the area surrounding the injury or incision. While this sounds wholly positive it is

never a reason to allow animals to suffer from postoperative pain where it can be avoided. The very hypersensitivity that is useful short term to protect the area reflects the changes in the central nervous system that contribute to 'wind-up' where short duration stimuli result in disproportionately longer periods of pain perception. Pre-emptive analgesia limits this effect and the clinician can take sensible measures to facilitate wound healing.

(2) *Chronic pain:* This is pain that persists beyond the expected time frame for a disease. Chronic pain is maladaptive, i.e. it has no biological function. All the components of acute pain that are so useful in the acute phase become part of the chronic disease process. It is vital that owners of animals in chronic pain understand this point. Acute pain, while undesirable and now avoidable to some extent because companion animals are not in the wild and can be looked after (therefore they do not need the survival advantage that acute pain gives them), is biologically useful, and sustains fitness and viability. It keeps animals alive. Chronic pain does none of those things, but one has to be alive to experience it.

Hypersensitivity

This phenomenon occurs in clinical pain and can be divided into peripheral and central sensitisation.

Peripheral sensitisation

This is mediated by chemical mediators such as substance P and calcitonin gene-related peptide (CGRP). These neurotransmitters, released after tissue damage, lower the response threshold for A delta and C fibres by creating a 'sensitising soup' of inflammatory cells and further mediators that act synergistically. This creates a zone of primary hyperalgesia around the original tissue injury.

Central sensitisation

'Wind-up' occurs when the synaptic action potentials generated by A delta and C fibres result in an increasing and long-lasting potentiation in dorsal horn neurons. It is mediated by N-methyl-D-aspartate (NMDA) receptors and effectively means that short periods (a few seconds) of C fibre input (such as a surgical incision) results in several minutes of pain transmission. In other words, although the procedure or injury may be of brief duration, the pain felt by the subject is always of longer duration. This 'wind-up' process is a normal physiological result of injury, but must be appreciated before pre-emptive analgesia can be effective.

Central sensitisation is often used synonymously with 'wind-up' but is distinct and may be regarded as more pathological. However, it is thought that if 'wind-up' can be controlled or limited central sensitisation is less likely to occur. It does not appear to be inevitable and is associated with secondary hyperalgesia (areas of hyperalgesia beyond the original injury), chronic pain syndromes and allodynia. It involves dynamic changes in dorsal horn neuron excitability, whereby the receptive fields of neurons are modified and afferent nerves other than A delta and C fibres, such as A beta fibres, are recruited. A beta mechanoreceptors are stimulated by touch and vibration, so, once recruited, generate the perception of pain as a result of these normally non-noxious stimuli.

Neuropathic pain

Neuropathic pain arises as a result of damage to the nervous system. In people it tends to be characterised by lancinating, burning, shooting type pains, which are often severe. Since no subjective description is available from the veterinary patient, the presence of neuropathic pain is deduced (undoubtedly sometimes incorrectly) from behaviour. Such behaviours include: jumping or starting as though having been stung, spinning round to look at or try to grab the area of the body perceived to be the cause, running away as though very frightened, the development of compulsive type disorders such as overgrooming, tail chasing or compulsive licking (although these disorders have other possible causes, both clinical and behavioural) pacing, digging or scraping at the floor as though trying to escape.

Neuropathic pain can arise as a result of abnormal central processing or abnormal peripheral input (direct damage to the nerves). Central sensitisation is a contributory factor to the clinical picture. It is a difficult type of pain to treat and usually requires pharmacological intervention with the use of medication such as tricyclic antidepressants or anticonvulsants. Acupuncture would not usually be regarded as the treatment of choice for this kind of pain, but, since one can never be sure of the actual source or nature of the pain in our veterinary species, it may be worth trying before progressing to more complex medication.

Sympathetically maintained pain

Sympathetically maintained pain is not well understood in man and is even more difficult to recognise in the veterinary species. It is not within the remit of this book to discuss the current state of the literature on these complex pains; suffice it to say that, in both neuropathic and sympathetically maintained pain, one would expect direct needling of the affected area to be difficult because of hyperalgesia and allodynia. One would also expect secondary postural and muscular changes that may well be amenable to acupuncture and contributing to the suffering, so, while not recommending acupuncture to treat these kinds of syndromes directly, there may be merit in using it as an adjunctive therapy.

Other effects of pain

These are numerous and are often summarised as 'the stress response', since clearly these changes may also occur with other unrelieved stressful stimuli such as fear. The changes are worth noting, since some animals in chronic pain may display some of these signs *only*. Improvements in signs such as excessive panting and fear responses can also be used to help measure the outcome of interventions (outcome measures):

- Increased sympathetic tone
- Vasoconstriction
- Increased heart rate
- Decreased gastrointestinal and urinary tone (changes in toileting patterns)
- Increased skeletal muscle tone (trembling and muscle fasciculation)
- Increases in cortisol, anti diruretic hormone (ADH), growth hormone (GH), etc.
- Catabolic state (weight loss with no other organic cause)
- Increased respiratory rate (panting in dogs, mouth breathing in cats)
- Fear and anxiety (sound sensitivity, anxiety around other dogs, for example)
- Increased blood viscosity
- Changes in sleep patterns, pacing and restlessness at night especially.

ASSESSING PAIN IN ANIMALS

In two surveys of UK veterinarians a significant proportion of practitioners indicated that one of the main reasons for withholding analgesia perioperatively was that they found it difficult to recognise when their patients were in pain[4]. Pain recognition, pain scoring systems, both acute and chronic, and pain management are areas of current research in veterinary schools.

Before pain can be recognised, the veterinarian needs to understand two main concepts: what pain is and how animals are likely to feel when in pain. The way animals feel determines the way that they will behave and behaviour is the key to pain recognition in our companion animal species.

The first part of this chapter has discussed what pain is and what it is for. It is worth reiterating here that the emotional or affective component of pain is what teaches an animal not to repeat a potentially damaging experience, either by avoiding a specific event or by guarding and resting the affected part.

If human subjects did not care about pain they would learn nothing useful from it and risk continued or repeated tissue damage. Caring about pain becomes a problem when that pain is chronic and therefore no longer 'useful'. Teaching patients to be in control of their pain and using drugs that remove the emotional component of pain (e.g. opiates: patients will still be aware of pain, but report that they no longer mind its presence) are two key methods of current pain management in humans.

Assessing pain by behavioural changes

When one considers more classical presentations of pain, e.g. limping, stiffness, it is in behavioural terms that their owners describe the pet's problems: reluctance to get up, lethargic, grumpy, hesitant to jump in the car, 'clingy', reluctant to play, etc. And it is in behavioural terms that the same owners describe an improvement in their pet's condition: more playful, keen to walk, less anxious, more puppy-like and so on.

Whether aware of it or not, veterinarians all tend to assess pain in animals by their behaviour, as well as by supposedly more objective measurements of pain and function such as percentage lameness, range of movements and the results of palpation and manipulation. Even these parameters are far more subjective than one would like to suppose and confounded by behavioural influences on the animals themselves. What is rarely considered when assessing an animal for pain is their motivation to perform certain behaviours. The drive to perform a given behaviour is influenced by internal and external factors, but what drives an animal is very different from what drives a human. Many dogs have a high motivation for exercise (especially collies and bull breeds) and will exercise apparently normally in the face of pain; therefore, exercising per se cannot be taken as evidence of lack of pain.

PAIN PRESENTING AS BEHAVIOUR PROBLEMS

Behaviour changes caused by pain include the three main categories that behaviourists recognise: aggression, anxiety and compulsive type behaviours[5]. Which behaviour might arise from pain in an individual is a result of the animal's individual temperament and the opportunities afforded by its environment, which of course include the interactions of people and other animals.

Aggression may arise directly as a result of pain being caused by a person or other animal. The animal may also be aggressive if it feels vulnerable to attack because of its condition, so status is likely to play a part in some pain-related behaviours in dogs, although fear will also be a component in other individuals and species. Severe pain may result in aggression whatever the status of the potential 'victim', but a lower intensity pain may only trigger aggression if the person or animal is of lower, equal or undetermined status.

Pain may be more likely to give rise to anxiety in timid individuals, because the animal's ability to cope with a given situation is diminished both physically and psychologically.

The most obvious compulsive behaviour arising from a pain is acral lick dermatitis (ALD)[6]. Local or referred pain of musculoskeletal or visceral origin can cause licking either to directly stimulate the site or as a displacement activity, both of which may become compulsive over time.

IDENTIFICATION OF PAIN

Identification of pain is not straightforward in non-human animals. A thorough musculoskeletal examination is mandatory, also bearing in mind the possibility that pain may be arising from abdominal or pelvic viscera and from dental problems.

The pain response in individuals will be different depending upon factors discussed above and dependent upon the examiner, but will include: startle, flinching, withdrawal and escape if possible, turning towards the painful area, attempting to bite or attack the perceived cause of pain, and vocalisation. Changes in facial expression, such as lip licking and ear movements, can also be noted.

Referred pain is difficult, if not impossible, to judge in animals, which makes identifying the site or origin of pain problematic. It should be remembered that painful conditions are not restricted to joints and bones – soft tissue pain can be significant, widespread and debilitating.

It should also be borne in mind that just because an animal is apparently sound does not mean it cannot have limb pain – bilateral hip dysplasia, for example, although one would expect an abnormal gait. Examination of muscles and soft tissue, particularly the muscles associated with the spine, should be detailed and attention paid to the site and response to palpation of myofascial trigger points which may indicate injury or trauma and which can, themselves, give rise to severe pain.

It should also be remembered that different examiners may elicit different responses from the same animal. This should not be surprising since it occurs for other types of handling. Different results from examination of the same animal may be due to a genuine difference in the animal's response to a different handler, a different environment in which the animal feels more, or less, relaxed, different palpation and examination techniques, differences in response with the owner present or absent and different intensities of pain experienced from one day, or hour, to the next.

This phenomenon highlights the need for repeatability of response elicited by the same examiner, especially if useful information is going to be obtained during and after treatment.

Pain in other species

When considering pain recognition in other species, the behaviour and natural history of that species should be taken into account. Just as the manifestation of pain in dogs can be influenced by motivation, position in the social hierarchy, breed traits and learned experiences, other species will display pain to a greater or lesser extent depending upon their ethology.

Prey species such as sheep and cattle are generally regarded to be 'stoical' because they will often continue to behave relatively normally in the face of pain. They will try to keep up with the flock or herd and they will not vocalise until the condition is too severe for this to be maintained. This behaviour does not occur because these species feel no pain, but because it is not in their interests to be obviously vulnerable. These species rely on their social groupings for management of resources and for safety; a lone animal is an obvious target for a predator, as is a vocalising one. Prey species that are better equipped to run, such as horses, will usually try to escape from a painful stimulus.

Pain in cats

Cats can be both a prey and predator, and may live as solitary or colony animals. Their response to pain appears to be highly complex and unpredictable. Pain is arguably more difficult to recognise convincingly in cats than in dogs and they are often more difficult to examine. Their high degree of reactivity to stimuli means that a response to palpation/examination is problematic to interpret. This should not be used as an excuse to avoid looking, however, or for not considering organic and dental, as well as musculoskeletal, origins of pain. Disc disease and osteoarthritis are now recognised as being more prevalent in cats than was previously supposed. Behavioural changes are the major indications of pain in this species. Cats are not regularly exercised by their owners so more obvious indications of pain, such as exercise intolerance, are often not picked up.

Pain in horses

Horses are a prey species whose usual response to an aversive stimulus is flight; aggression is likely to occur if escape is thwarted. Although they arguably have a more profound learned response to a one-off painful event than do dogs and cats, it should not be assumed that reaction to palpation, saddling, or manipulation is merely a learned behaviour. It has been discussed in depth by Casey[7], that horses are just as likely, if not more so given the demands made upon them by man, to suffer from chronic, intermittent painful conditions, particularly of the musculoskeletal system, which will give rise to unpredictable and apparently irrational behaviour[5].

Pain in reptiles, birds and amphibians

From the neurophysiological studies performed on reptiles there is no reason to believe that pain perception in these species differs in any significant way from mammalian species. Their response to a potentially painful stimulus is similar to that of any animal species: startle, withdrawal and escape if possible, turning towards the painful area, attempting to bite or attack the perceived cause of pain, 'vocalisation' in terms of hissing, spitting and jaw plate grinding (turtles).

Summary

(1) Acute pain including surgical pain should be treated or pre-empted effectively to minimise suffering, wind-up and possible chronic pain syndromes associated with central sensitisation.

(2) Chronic pain is a disease in itself and has no biological function.

(3) There are four distinct components to pain. The affective component represents suffering and can be targeted and influenced separately from the others, although ideally all four would be addressed. However, positive behavioural changes in mood and activity without obvious gait changes or increased range of joint movement may indicate reduction in suffering without significant reduction in the sensory component.

(4) This means that *all* possible outcome measures should be considered when assessing the merits of any intervention.

REFERENCES

1. Pain terms: a current list with definitions and notes on usage. In: Merskey H, Bogduk N, editors. *Classification of Chronic Pain: Descriptions of Chronic Pain Syndromes and Definitions of Pain Terms*, 2nd edn. Seattle: IASP Press; 1994. pp. 209–14.

2. Lamont LA, Tranquilli WJ, Grimm KA. Physiology of pain. *Vet Clin North Am Small Anim Pract* 2000;30(4):703–28.

3. Bonica JJ. *The Management of Pain*. Philadelphia: Lea & Febiger; 1953. pp. 141–42.

4. Capner CA, Lascelles BD, Waterman-Pearson AE. Current British veterinary attitudes to perioperative analgesia for dogs. *Vet Rec* 1999;145(4):95–9.

5. Scott S. Clinical causes of behaviour problems. *Proceedings of the Association of Veterinary Teachers and Research Workers* 1999;49.

6. Veith L. Acral lick dermatitis in the dog. *Canine Pract* 1974;13(1):15–22.

7. Casey RA. Pain induced behavioural problems – clinical cases. *Proceedings of the 38th British Equine Veterinary Association* 1999;22.

The use of acupuncture for musculoskeletal pain

SOURCES OF PAIN IN MUSCULOSKELETAL PROBLEMS

Osteoarthritis

This condition is a progressive degenerative disease of synovial joints. It is characterised by pain, disability, destruction of articular cartilage and bony remodelling. Inflammation of the synovial membrane creates further destruction and inflammation and it is this synovitis that is thought to be the source of much of the pain of osteoarthritis, although it can be difficult to demonstrate inflammatory cells in joint fluid.

Disc related pain

The sources of pain related to disc herniation are not completely understood. To some extent the muscle spasm and myofascial trigger points set up by the acute pain of disc rupture are secondary and more thoroughly understood, but the pain derived from disc herniation itself is not so well comprehended. A study in 2003 assessed changes in brain-derived neurotrophic factor (BDNF) expression[1], a modulator of nociceptive information, in the dorsal root ganglion (DRG) and spinal cord dorsal horn following experimental disc herniation. According to this study, immunohistochemical analysis revealed an increase in percentage of BDNF-immunoreactive (IR) neurons profiles in the affected DRG and marked elevation in the BDNF-IR regions within both the superficial and deep layers at the corresponding spinal level with a peak at three days after nucleus pulposus (NP)

79

application. These results therefore show that herniated NP increases the BDNF production in the pain-processing neurons. The conclusion of this study is that such changes can contribute to the development of inflammatory hyperalgesia.

Neuropathic pain

This is not musculoskeletal in origin, but is included here because it may present as such and its effects may cause secondary pain and dysfunction in muscle. Neuropathic pain arises from direct damage to the nerves and characteristically presents as lancinating, burning, sharp or shooting pain. Since animals cannot verbalise what they feel, it must be inferred from their behaviour. Sudden jumping, starting, turning around and attacking various parts of the body are the kinds of signs seen with neuropathic and disc related pain. Overgrooming in cats and so-called 'feline hyperaesthesia syndrome' may also be signs of such pain in individual cases. These signs are not pathognomic, but *suggestive* of neuropathic pain.

Muscle pain

Any musculoskeletal condition will cause subtle to gross changes in posture and balance. These will affect other joints and muscle groups, causing strain (trigger points), further wear and tear on the joints, shortening and weakening of the muscles. Muscles may also atrophy, causing more pressure to be placed on functional muscles.

Classically, dogs with hip arthritis will throw more weight onto their forequarters, exacerbating elbow and shoulder problems. Their epaxial muscles are also predictably painful on palpation, presumably because they are using them to compensate for the drive and manoeuvrability lost from the hindquarters.

MYOFASCIAL TRIGGER POINTS

Definitions

- **Myofascial pain:** Pain arising from an active myofascial trigger point.
- **Myofascial pain syndrome:** The sensory, motor and autonomic symptoms caused by myofascial trigger points[2].
- **Myofascial trigger point:** A myofascial trigger point is defined as a hyperirritable locus within a taut band of skeletal muscle or its

associated fascia. It is painful on compression and can evoke a characteristic referral pattern of pain or autonomic dysfunction. It may exhibit a jump sign or twitch response[3].

In other words, a trigger point is a tender point in a taut band of muscle that can cause referred pain. Firm palpation across the taut band of a trigger point can result in an involuntary jerk by the subject: this is the **jump sign**. At the same time the taut band is sometimes seen or felt to contract briefly: this is the **local twitch response**.

A selected historical view

In the East, the observation and treatment of trigger points probably arose alongside the earliest development of acupuncture techniques. In traditional Chinese medicine (TCM) there are points known as *ah shi* points. *Ah shi* is a phrase roughly equivalent to 'oh, yes!' – an exclamation taken to indicate that the palpation of a tender point has located the patient's pain. The phrase usually accompanies the involuntary jerk known as the jump sign. *Ah shi* points were then used as part of the point selection process and needled. The points that were frequently identified as *ah shi* points were incorporated into the nomenclature of acupuncture and are given names as acupuncture points. Not surprisingly, and although an *ah shi* point is not always directly equivalent to a trigger point, the location of trigger points often correlates precisely with that of acupuncture points[4], and their associated referral patterns sometimes describe a strikingly similar path to the meridian. To illustrate this the following exercise is suggested.

Grip the upper free border of trapezius between fingers and thumb, as illustrated in Figure 6.1. Find the taut band that is uncomfortable on pressure (in man, there is almost always one in this position) and then press harder. Sustain the pressure until you can feel the pain referring. The classical referral pattern is up the side of the neck to the ear, as shown in Figure 6.2, or even around the side of the head to the temple. (Failure to elicit any referral pattern indicates not enough pressure is being applied!) This trigger point coincides exactly with the position of an acupuncture point called GB21 (GB standing for Gall Bladder – the name of the meridian on which this point is found). The Gall Bladder meridian is said to run in the pattern shown in Figure 6.3, over the side of the head – reminiscent of the characteristic pattern of referred pain from the trigger point. Although it is hardly proof, and some evidence suggests that the notion of

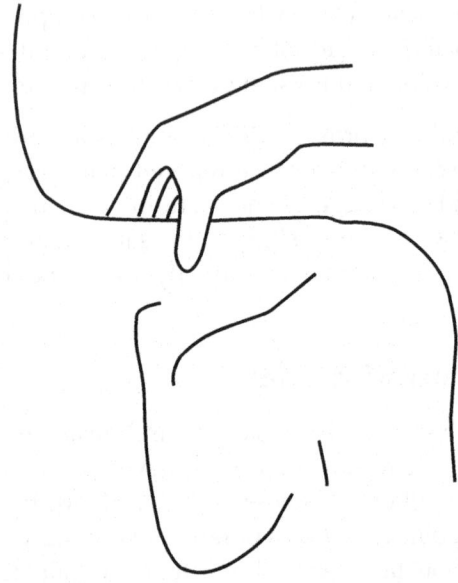

Figure 6.1 The pincer grip on the upper trapezius muscle in humans.

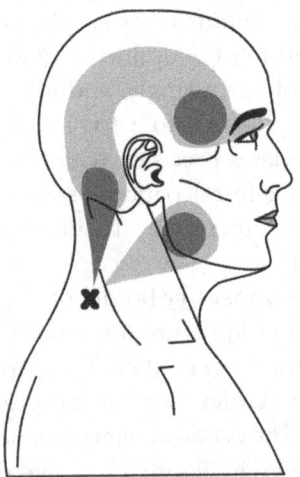

Figure 6.2 Referral pattern from myofascial trigger point in the upper trapezius muscle.

meridians existed before that of acupoints; it is possible that the courses of some of the meridians were described because of the patterns of pain consistently described by patients when the points were pressed or needled.

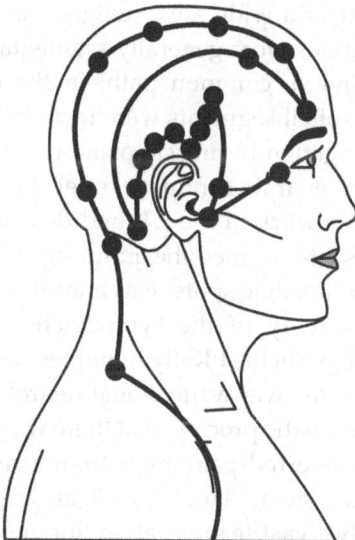

Figure 6.3 The gall bladder meridian, showing similarity of path of meridian over the head and the referral pattern from the trigger point in upper trapezius, which coincides with the point GB or Gall Bladder 21.

It can be difficult for physicians and veterinarians to grasp that such an apparently important phenomenon as the trigger point (its importance will be described later) could exist without their having been taught about it during their training. One of the main reasons for this is the plethora of names given to these points since they were first observed in the West. Such terms as 'muscle callouses'[5], 'muscular rheumatism'[6], 'myitis chronica rheumatica'[7], 'myogelosis'[8], and 'muscle hardenings'[9] were the forerunners to the term 'fibrositis', which was introduced by Gowers in 1904[10]. The latter term has survived in common use until surprisingly recently, considering that inflammation of connective tissue has never been consistently and reliably demonstrated in biopsy studies. In other words there is no '-itis' involved and the main problem arises from muscle not from fibrous tissue. This is quite a misnomer to have survived so long. However, in 1938, having noted the pain referral patterns described by some of his patients with tender muscle nodules, Kellgren investigated the pain referral patterns produced by injecting hypertonic saline into the muscles and other soft tissues of experimental subjects, and in true scientific spirit, subjected himself to many such procedures[11]. In muscle he found that pain was more diffuse than in other soft tissues, and that as the stimulus intensified the pain pattern could spread over a wide area. Kellgren and his peers concluded that the distributions were generally segmental, but recognised that the pain must have a 'common path' in the central nervous system when several spinal segments were included.

Investigation of muscle pain syndromes continued independently on three separate continents after these discoveries. Good continued Kellgren's work in the UK and described the patient's pain reaction that was later termed the 'jump sign'. He felt that the process responsible for 'myalgic spots' was a local constriction of blood vessels due to overactivity of the sympathetic nerves supplying them[12]. The Australian Michael Kelly hypothesised that the phenomenon known as 'fibrositis' was a functional neurological disturbance caused by a local rheumatic process, that there was little or no local pathology and that the referred pain arose from a reflex disturbance of the central nervous system[13]. Janet Travell, an American physician and one of J.F. Kennedy's vast team of attending medics, devoted her career to the study of 'myofascial trigger points'. She initially emphasised the importance of the referral pattern from the trigger point and postulated that any fibroblastic proliferation was secondary to a functional disorder, with pathological changes occurring only if the condition existed for a long time. She went on to develop the concept that the self-sustaining characteristic of trigger points depended on a feedback mechanism between the trigger points and the central nervous system[14]. Latterly she collaborated with Simons to produce a comprehensive manual covering the field of myofascial pain. These tomes are standard literature for any physician with an interest in muscle pain and dysfunction in man.

Pathophysiology of myofascial trigger points

There have been numerous attempts to cut out trigger points and demonstrate histologically that there is some tangible pathology to account for the taut band and knotty feel of these loci. These have consistently failed and this is another reason why the concept of myofascial pain has not been readily incorporated into veterinary and medical training. One study did succeed in demonstrating a difference between muscle cells from patients with fibromyalgia (a chronic pain syndrome, probably centrally mediated, but of unknown aetiology, but recognised to give rise to multiple, bilaterally sensitive trigger points in sufferers) and those with chronic myofascial pain[15].

Gerwin notes that, despite years of clinical study, the pathophysiology of the trigger point has remained elusive[16], but, thanks to Hubbard and Berkoff, there is now electromyographic evidence supporting the presence of at least a functional abnormality at the trigger point[17]. There have been several negative electromyographic studies of trigger points over the last 30 years, including Durette *et al.*[18], but in 1993 Hubbard and Berkoff demonstrated increased electrical activity within an area of 1–2 mm around the trigger point relative to a normal area of the same muscle. This finding has been repeated many times since, and, importantly, Couppé *et al.* provided a blinded correlation between the clinical location of trigger points and increased electrical activity in muscle[19]. Essentially, these studies demonstrated that the insertion of an EMG needle at a trigger point gave significantly higher readings of spontaneous electrical activity (SEA) than did insertion of an EMG needle close by in the same muscle at two locations that were also acupuncture points. Hubbard and Berkoff continued this work in cooperation with McNulty and Gervirtz and showed that a psychological stressor significantly increased the electrical activity of trapezius trigger points compared with a non-stressful control task[20]. So there is a potential pathophysiological marker for the trigger points, and the suggestion that it is influenced by stress-induced autonomic activity.

There was some debate regarding the site of origin of the SEA in the muscles. It was proposed by Hubbard and Berkoff that SEA derived from the intrafusal fibres of muscle spindles[21], but more recently Hong and Simons have put forward a strong argument in favour of dysfunctional motor endplates[22].

The argument runs as follows: motor endplates normally release acetylcholine (ACh) in sufficient quantities to depolarise nerves and cause muscle contraction. When these endplates are dysfunctional, either with age, pathology or direct damage (such as blunt trauma to the muscle), they leak small amounts of ACh. This is not enough to cause muscle contraction, but sufficient to cause 'bunching' of the sarcomeres in the region of the endplate. This bunching is what gives rise to the characteristic taut band. Physical restriction on the blood vessels in this area of the muscle compromises their ability to remove the toxic waste products of muscle metabolism. These products accumulate locally and sensitise the local sensory nerves. Because these nerves are now more sensitive, the region within the band is now 'hyperirritable' and this gives rise to the characteristic tender spot. The local twitch response (LTR), which is sometimes seen when the band is plucked or needled, represents the release of sufficient ACh to cause contraction in the local fibres.

Classification of trigger points

Myofascial trigger points can be classified as follows:

(1) An **active** trigger point causes a clinical pain complaint. Trigger points can be found in most adults over 25 years of age as a result of degeneration. Dogs older than one year of age are likely to have developed some trigger points (personal observation, SL). Just because a trigger point, with all its characteristics, is found does not mean that it is causing the patient any discomfort at any time other than when it is palpated. A trigger point must be active to be clinically relevant.

(2) A **latent** trigger point does not cause spontaneous pain, but is painful on compression and causes some restriction of movement. In animals, the greatest challenge is to judge which trigger points are active and which latent. Unfortunately, it is either a matter of clinical experience and extensive palpation practice to be able to judge which trigger points are likely to be causing the problem in an individual, or it is largely guesswork. The relevance of latent trigger points is twofold: first the restriction of movement may be problematic in athletes, such as the competition horse or racing greyhound. Second, the presence of latent trigger points is a potential source of an apparently disproportionate amount of pain following injury – when multiple latent trigger points may become active.

(3) A **primary** trigger point is activated directly by some form of mechanical trauma to the skeletal muscle in which it occurs. It is the cause of the clinical signs and if treated successfully those signs should completely resolve. A muscle strain may create a primary, active trigger point.

(4) A **secondary** trigger point develops as a result of the dysfunction of a primary trigger point, or secondary to the pain or dysfunction caused by other somatic or visceral pathology. For example, trigger points are commonly found in the triceps muscles of dogs with elbow osteoarthritis. These trigger points are secondary to the joint pathology.

(5) A **satellite** trigger point is a secondary trigger point that develops in the pain reference zone from a primary trigger point, or the pain reference zone from other somatic or visceral pathology. The relevance of this in animals is not clear, since we cannot be certain of pain referral patterns. However, for example, if a trigger point

were set up in the infraspinatus muscle secondary to shoulder arthritis and the pain from that trigger point were referred down the lateral aspect of the forelimb (as it is in humans), then a satellite trigger point may be set up in the triceps muscle.

Prevalence of trigger points in man

Myofascial trigger points are recognised by many clinicians to be one of the most common causes of pain and dysfunction in the musculoskeletal system. In UK general practice it has been estimated that up to 20% of consultations result from myofascial pain[23]. Trigger points have been detected in the shoulder girdle musculature in nearly half of a group of young, asymptomatic military personnel[24], and with a similar prevalence in the masticatory muscles of a group of unselected student nurses. Active trigger points, those causing spontaneous pain, have been diagnosed as the primary source of pain in 74% of 96 patients with musculoskeletal pain seen by a neurologist in a community pain medical centre[25], and in 85% of 283 consecutive admissions to a comprehensive pain centre[26]. Of 164 patients referred to a dental clinic for chronic head and neck pain 55% were found to have active myofascial trigger points as the cause of their pain[27], as were 30% of those presenting with pain to a university primary care internal medicine group practice from a consecutive series of 172 patients[28]. A recent study of musculoskeletal disorders in villagers from rural Thailand has demonstrated myofascial pain as the primary diagnosis in 36% of 431 subjects with pain during the previous seven days[29]. In other words myofascial pain is a significant cause of pain and suffering in humans.

Aetiology

Travell and Simons put forward three aetiological factors responsible for the development of primary trigger points: acute physical overload (muscle strain), overwork fatigue (such as postural) and chilling (sitting in a draft!). They also describe trigger points developing secondarily to some other pathological process or event. Their assertions are supported only by empirical evidence, and how such factors may cause the development of trigger points is the subject of much speculation. In the second edition of *The Trigger Point Manual* Simons no longer lists chilling as an aetiological factor, but adds radiculopathy and gross trauma[2]. In animals, muscle strain may be seen in athletes, such as the competition horse or racing greyhound, or as a result of an enthusiastic chase, a sudden twist or encounter with a rabbit hole. Postural overwork fatigue may not seem an obvious aetiological factor in animals since they do not slump over computer keyboards or steering wheels, but dogs that pull on the lead consistently appear to have more sensitive trigger points in caudal trapezius muscles and those that throw their weight forward to compensate for pain or dysfunction in their hindquarters appear to develop trigger points in the muscles of the lumbar spine without any local pathology (personal observations, SL).

Clinical features

The most common presenting feature of a trigger point is pain. Myofascial pain is deep, dull and aching in nature, but can vary tremendously in severity and presentation. As it increases in severity there is more likely to be a wide referral pattern and it is not uncommon for the patient to be completely unaware of its site of origin. The referral pattern of pain is often characteristic of the muscle of origin, but some individuals appear to be more likely to develop distant referral than others. The veterinarian should be alert to the possibility of a distant trigger point when presented with signs such as licking of the distal limbs, as well as the more obvious possibility of neuropathic pain. The pain can be exacerbated by stretching or contraction of the muscle that contains the active trigger point. This can be manifest as an acute exacerbation of pain with movement or can develop more insidiously at rest, particularly in bed at night when the muscle concerned is left in a shortened position, or under slight tension. Restlessness and agitation are common manifestations of pain in dogs and are often worse at night when, presumably, they are used to being more settled. For man, massage, hot baths and showers can relieve the pain, particularly if followed by stretching of the specific muscle concerned. In animals, stretching of the muscles is also used, especially after they have been warmed up by exercise or massage. It should be noted that flat hand massage is preferable in animals unless one is specifically trying to treat the trigger point by digital pressure (and this is not to be recommended to owners). Poking and prodding trigger points in an attempt to mimic the kinds of massage the owner might appreciate for their own sore muscles may result in an exacerbation of pain.

Burning and lancinating pains are less commonly associated with trigger points, however, paraesthesia ('pins and needles') in the absence of real sensory disturbance can frequently be associated.

In treating human patients, one should beware of those who have symmetrical trigger points and bilateral symptoms. Myofascial pain syndromes are rarely symmetrical. These patients may have, or be developing, fibromyalgia[30]. Such patients may have subtle abnormalities of sensory processing, and vigorous direct needling of their trigger points may not be the optimum therapeutic intervention. In the veterinary literature, Jansenns makes reference to some of his patients, in a case series describing the identification and treatment of trigger points, as having bilaterally symmetrical trigger points and not responding to treatment. He concludes that these animals 'may have fibromyalgia'[31]. It is important to note that fibromyalgia has not been demonstrated in animals and that there is more to this condition than multiple trigger points. It is not uncommon to find apparently bilaterally symmetrical trigger points in animals, but the pain response elicited from each side should be different. In other words it is the pain that is usually unilateral, not the trigger points, and it is difficult to be confident that one is putting as much pressure on one side as the other.

Clinical findings

Examination of a trigger point in man should reveal a tender point in a taut band of muscle, i.e. a tender knot of muscle. Pressure over this point is likely to reproduce the patient's symptoms, and as the examiner's fingers are drawn across the tender point of the band (like slowly plucking the string of a guitar) the patient will jerk involuntarily (the 'jump sign'), withdrawing slightly from the examiner's hand. The patient often utters a brief exclamation as they jump – Oh yes! That's it! Ouch yes! Even patients not familiar with the correct Chinese expression are occasionally heard to utter something like *ah shi*. In superficial muscles it is possible to see the taut band twitch when performing this manoeuvre: the 'local twitch response'. In animals, it is impossible to tell whether or not one has elicited the patient's pain. All that can be inferred is that the points hurt: a dog's reaction will be anything from the 'jump sign' to yelping and turning to snap (or in the case of a typical labrador: more vigorous tail wagging!); horses may move away or try to kick or stamp; cats may startle, hiss, scratch or try to escape. The price of success in finding a trigger point in an animal usually involves a finely honed sense of survival.

Needling can be useful diagnostically, especially when it is difficult to feel a taut band or see a local twitch response. The human patient is more likely to feel referred pain on needling the trigger point than on digital compression. In humans and animals the local twitch response can often be felt more easily than it is seen.

Muscle harbouring an active trigger point is invariably slightly shortened. This will result in restriction of the full range of motion in directions that fully elongate the muscle. Muscle shortening can be a very useful sign in some areas of the body, and less useful in others. An active trigger point in the cranial trapezius muscle will result in a restriction of lateral neck flexion to the same side. If particularly severe, there will be restriction of flexion to the opposite side as well. Treatment should restore full movement provided that there is no concurrent restriction of axial structures.

It is not uncommon for trigger points to appear to move during the course of treatment. They do not move, but as satellite trigger points are deactivated, active trigger points are uncovered closer to the original source of pain or injury.

In humans, trigger points are most often found in the postural muscles of the neck, shoulders and pelvic girdle. Sedentary people in their middle years present most commonly with the pain of active trigger points. Women present for treatment more commonly than men, and it is not clear whether this is due to a greater prevalence of myofascial pain in women, or to confounding factors that affect consultation rates.

In animals it is assumed that trigger points can be found in any muscle, but the majority of them appear to be found in similar muscle groups. This is partly because these muscles are under the greatest strain, but also that they are associated with common orthopaedic problems.

The guiding principles for searching for trigger points are:

(1) Search in the areas of the species' musculature under the greatest biomechanical strain during normal activity.
(2) Search in the areas most subject to degenerative disease, e.g. if this species tends to suffer with arthritis of the hip, look for secondary trigger points in the hip girdle musculature.

In the individual animal:

(3) Search in the areas subject to the greatest biomechanical strain resulting from unique behaviour exhibited by the animal, or its owner, e.g. in trapezius muscles of dogs who pull on the lead.
(4) Search in areas at risk due to environmental factors peculiar to the animal's individual circumstances.

Examination of muscle for trigger points

There are two main techniques used for palpating skeletal muscle for trigger points. The most universally applicable is flat palpation perpendicular to the direction of the muscle fibres. The muscle is placed on a slight stretch and the examining fingers indent the skin over the muscle and palpate firmly to and fro across a short distance so that skin moves with the fingers across the muscle fibres. It is not always possible to put the muscles to be examined on a slight stretch in animals, so the taut 'band' may feel more like a 'knot'. The examining hand is then moved a short distance further across the muscle, and the process is repeated. The other method is the pincer grip technique. This can only be applied to certain muscles, particularly those with free borders such as trapezius, sternocleidomastoid and pectoralis major in man; in triceps, rectus femoris, semimembranosus and semitendinosus in dogs and cats. The 'pincer' is formed between the thumb and forefinger or middle finger, and is applied to an edge or fold of muscle. The fibres are allowed to slip between the fingertip and thumb as the hand is drawn away perpendicular to the direction of the fibres. The muscle needs to be more relaxed for this technique than for flat palpation.

Reliability of clinical diagnosis

There have been several studies testing the inter-observer reliability of examining for trigger points. Those using untrained examiners failed to demonstrate reliability[32, 33]. The most recent study, using experienced clinicians, demonstrated reliability in its second phase after the examiners underwent a three-hour period of training[34]. This training period was aimed at developing consensus on interpretation of physical signs, rather than training the clinicians in how to find trigger points. The following clinical features tested are placed in order of overall interrater reliability from the results of the latter study:

(1) Pain recognition
(2) Taut band
(3) Tender point
(4) Referred pain
(5) Local twitch response.

This study has been repeated as far as it is possible to do so at Glasgow University Veterinary School. The results are not yet available but tend to reiterate the need for clinicians experienced in palpating trigger points in animals. The greatest difficulty with this study is the absence of the most reliable sign: pain recognition. Without pain recognition, the presence of a taut band must be agreed upon before deciding whether a pain response and local twitch are present.

Many veterinarians have been taught to find trigger points and use the palpation techniques in their diagnosis and treatment of musculoskeletal problems. This does not prove that they are all finding trigger points or would all find the same features in the same place, but for now is the best that can be achieved.

Treatment of trigger points

The physical modalities most frequently applied to treat trigger points are pressure and stretch. Dry needling is undoubtedly one of the most effective methods of applying pressure to discrete areas of tissue, and in combination with specific muscle stretching appears to be a very efficient method of rehabilitating patients with troublesome or recurrent myofascial pain. Injection techniques are often applied to trigger points: this technique is frequently used in the US by veterinarians, but is not so common in the UK. A variety of different substances are used for injection, such as water, vitamin B12, botulinum toxin (more common in medical practice) and, most popularly, local anaesthetics. The idea is that the substance will continue to stimulate the trigger point and thereby maintain the effect. However, clinical studies indicate that dry needling is no different from injection therapy (wet needling) in terms of efficacy[35–37]. When wet needling is used it does not seem to matter what is injected[38]. The logical conclusion from these findings is that it is the needle which is mediating the effect[39]. However, it is possible that the needle is simply acting as a very powerful placebo. Further research is needed to determine the specific effect (i.e. the effect beyond placebo) of direct needling on myofascial trigger point pain.

A host of non-needling therapies are applied to trigger points, but discussion of these is of less relevance in a text on acupuncture. Animal physiotherapists use digital pressure (so-called 'acupressure', although no needle is involved) and this can be effective; but for some patients this is too painful and it is not always possible to achieve enough pressure to deactivate the trigger point without an adverse reaction from the patient.

Prognosis

Simple clinical audit suggests that the majority of human patients get better with dry needling[40]. This is more difficult to say for animals, because by the time they are presented for acupuncture many have been suffering from multiple painful problems for many months, if not years. In these cases, the clinician will not be treating only trigger points. However, as veterinary acupuncture becomes more widely used in general practice and more clinicians start to look for and treat primary trigger points, then audit will be possible.

As a general rule, myofascial pain syndromes that have been present for six months or less in human patients appear to be curable, but those that have been present longer, or have followed a chronic relapsing course, can only be treated symptomatically, with a latent tendency to relapse remaining (White, personal communication 1994). Again, further audit is required on the treatment of primary trigger points in animals to be able to compare these observations. When treating trigger points secondary to a condition such as osteoarthritis, it is expected that the trigger points will be reactivated in time because of local joint pain and postural changes.

If the patient is not significantly improved after, say, two or three sessions, the therapist must consider the possibility that:

(1) The primary trigger point has not been correctly identified and treated.
(2) The diagnosis of myofascial pain syndrome is incorrect.
(3) There are factors causing persistence of the treated trigger point that have been overlooked.

If the initial assessment has been performed by an experienced clinician, the last point is the most likely cause of treatment failure. Persistent biomechanical stress is likely to be the most prevalent factor, but psychological stress with increased muscle tension is also possible in animals, although not as common as in humans. Dogs with sound sensitivities ('noise phobia') frequently have painful trigger points in their epaxial muscles (observation, SL). It can be difficult to decide whether the trigger points have arisen secondarily to chronic tension and fear or whether there is an underlying painful condition that is actually contributing to or causing the sound sensitivity.

Less common factors causing persistence of trigger points have been identified as borderline hypothyroidism[41] and other endocrine, metabolic and nutritional inadequacies in man. There is no reason to suppose that these factors would not be relevant in animals. Any condition that delays normal healing may predispose to the formation and maintenance of trigger points. While these factors have been suggested by empirical observation and remain to be validated, a working knowledge of the most common is essential to clinicians treating myofascial pain.

Trigger points in animals – specific comments

While members of the medical profession may sometimes feel it would be advantageous if their patients could not speak, the absence of verbal clues in animal patients is certainly a disadvantage when determining pain recognition, areas of pain, or pain referral patterns. As previously discussed, one of the most reliable features of an active trigger point is the ability to reproduce the patient's symptoms (usually pain) by pressing on it. Clearly, determining the precise nature of an animal's pain is impossible, so those features found to be most reliable in identifying trigger points in humans cannot be automatically applied to other animals.

The 'jump sign' often represents a physical correlate of 'pain recognition'. There is an involuntary jerk of the whole body, which is probably a brainstem reflex to the pain resulting from mechanical stimulation of a sufficiently active trigger point. In humans it is often associated with an exclamation of recognition, hence the *ah shi* point. Local tenderness is a necessary prerequisite for diagnosing a trigger point, but it is not specific. Tenderness can be assumed from behaviour, although this can vary dramatically due to factors such as the animal's temperament. Even 'nice' dogs can bite if one inadvertently presses a very active trigger point a little too hard and cats tend to give the clinician limited chances to repeat their mistakes.

Taut bands can only be felt with confidence in superficial muscles, and local twitch responses appear to vary greatly in their inter-observer reliability dependent on the site of the trigger point. In certain muscles, such as trapezius, a local twitch will result in a dramatic movement of the overlying skin and fascia, presumably due to the fact that skin and associated structures are much more mobile over the body of an animal than man. This is distinct from, and should not be confused with, the panniculus reflex in response to cutaneous stimulation.

So, we are left with fewer useful signs of trigger points for application in animals than we can apply to man. Are there others that we can consider that have not been tested for reliability in man? Trigger points invariably cause shortening of the affected muscle, and may cause a loss of power without muscle atrophy. Muscle shortening results in decreased range of movement (ROM) of the associated joint or joints. This can be a very helpful sign, but its usefulness is determined by how easy it is to measure the relevant ROM in a clinical setting. The clinical evaluation of power is not a reliable technique in the assessment of trigger points in humans, however, it is possible that in other animals it could be worthwhile: force plate studies may help to determine this point.

In summary, the following features may be useful in determining the presence of trigger points in animals:

- Taut band
- Jump sign
- Local tenderness
- Decreased ROM
- Local twitch response
- Decreased power.

Summary of myofascial trigger points in animals

(1) There is less certainty about the relevance of trigger points in animals than in humans because there has been less work done in this field.

(2) Muscle physiology in mammals is similar, so there is every reason to suppose that trigger points are present and relevant in non-human animals.

(3) Veterinarians and animal physiotherapists trained in finding trigger points locate and treat these entities frequently.

(4) Experimental work on trigger points is done using animal models, in particular the biceps femoris muscle of the rabbit[42].

(5) Clinically, they appear to be found in those muscles that bear the greatest biomechanical strain.

(6) Clinical observation indicates that most dogs over one year of age will develop trigger points in the caudal trapezius muscles as 'normal' wear and tear. Judging the clinical relevance of these becomes a matter of clinical experience: i.e. balancing the pain response with the primary source of pain and comparisons with animals without clinical signs.

(7) Any veterinarian wishing to become experienced in the diagnosis and treatment of trigger points should practise palpating for them in all animals of the species they wish to treat, so that it is

easier to distinguish between those trigger points that are latent and those that are active. This is important because: (a) many animals will have multiple trigger points and it may not be practical to treat them all; and (b) needling or digital pressure on a latent trigger point may cause it to become temporarily active and the animal's signs will worsen rather than improve.

(8) Trigger points can produce symptoms that appear to be much more severe than would be expected from the injury sustained by the patient or given the absence of bony changes on radiography. It is reported that, in man, a trivial injury can produce severe myofascial pain in a patient who has a number of latent trigger points waiting to be activated. These latent trigger points may have been set up after previous injuries or gradually developed from chronic overuse, but remained subclinical. Such a collection of latent trigger points can be referred to as an 'injury pool', and a relatively minor insult can activate them all at once, thus producing pain disproportionate to the severity of the injury. This appears to be the case in animals too: arthritic patients who have been stable for some time present with sudden worsening of their signs that may prompt a reinvestigation of their joint pathology. If there is no evidence of change here, one should look to the likelihood of myofascial pain having been triggered by an event such as a mild twist to the limb, or even just going for a slightly longer walk (dogs), or being exercised more vigorously than usual (horses).

ROLE OF ACUPUNCTURE IN TREATING MUSCULOSKELETAL PAIN

Osteoarthritis

There is evidence of specific efficacy (i.e. an effect beyond placebo) of acupuncture in the treatment of knee osteoarthritis in humans[43–45]. From a neurophysiological perspective the pain of osteoarthritis is likely to be best treated by a segmental approach. The aim is to inhibit the pain of synovitis by competing with it at the dorsal horn of the spinal segment for the affected joint. In effect, this means needling as close to the source of pain as possible, without entering the joint space. Although the chance of causing joint infection in this way is small, it would be disastrous for the joint concerned. For the same reason, metallic prostheses should also not be needled.

In practice, the structures needled are: acupuncture points close to the affected joint; muscles surrounding the joint, particularly those that are tender or have trigger points; periosteum at the joint margins ('periosteal pecking'); trigger points that appear active in the muscles associated with the joint; trigger points and tender points in muscles that may be under biomechanical strain because of postural changes. Clinical audit (SL) estimates a 70–80% chance of improvement in dogs with osteoarthritic pain. That improvement may be anything from a mild improvement in mobility to a dramatic improvement in demeanour and activity.

Myofascial pain syndromes

Here the pain of trigger points is treated by directly needling the trigger point. The mechanism of action is not known, but it may be through a spinal reflex mechanism similar to that which mediates the local twitch response, or it may simply be an example of segmental pain modulation.

Disc-related pain and neuropathic pain

These are notoriously difficult kinds of pain to treat successfully. Pain that is genuinely arising from the effects of a prolapsed disc may only be relieved by surgical decompression or other intervention. However, it is likely that with chronic conditions other structures are involved in the overall pain picture. One can predictably find trigger points associated with chronic disc prolpase, although it is by no means certain that the disc prolapse caused the trigger points to be activated. A painful prolapse is likely to set up trigger points, and after the condition has settled down it is possible that the majority of the patient's pain is arising from the trigger points and not the disc. Chronic pain, with signs of disc disease but without neurological signs, may well be worth treating with acupuncture. Acute spinal pain with neurological signs or associated with areas that do not reliably give rise to neurological signs (cats generally, cervical discs in dogs) should always be referred for a neurological work-up. Acupuncture is clearly not an appropriate treatment for acute disc prolapse with cord compression. However, some papers suggest that acupuncture may have a role to play in the very early treatment of spinal cord injury[46-48]. The studies looked at experimental spinal cord injuries and the effects of early electroacupuncture treatment. The first, in rats, showed improved function in those rats who had been treated 15 minutes post-injury compared with those that received no treatment; there was also a minimisation of post-injury spinal-cord shrinkage and a marked sparing of ventral horn neurons. The second, in cats, suggested that an increase in acid phosphatase levels in the treated groups may improve regeneration in the recovery period. These are experimental papers and may not correlate usefully with the clinical picture of injury. However, it appears to be necessary in any case to intervene early and for most practical purposes this is unlikely to occur, especially as the injured animal is likely to be undergoing other life-saving treatments even if it reaches a clinic within the critical time.

Neuropathic pain is not straightforward to diagnose, especially in non-human animals. It is problematic to treat, although tricyclic anti-depressants and some anticonvulsants appear useful in this regard. Acupuncture may be useful too, perhaps because the signs of muscular or myofascial pain have confused the picture and are in fact the major causes of pain, although relieving some secondary muscular discomfort would be helpful in any case. Neuropathic pain problems frequently result in patient's showing signs of hyperalgesia and allodynia; i.e. they have a disproportionate response to peripheral stimuli, which they perceive as more aversive than usual. This central sensitisation may be effectively damped down by sequential acupuncture treatments (via upregulation of inhibitory mechanisms). However, it is important to note that in this case, needling close to the source of pain may not be appropriate. Acupuncture usually stimulates A delta or type III nerve fibres and stimulation of these does not produce aversive feelings. Because of the change in perception of peripheral stimuli, a needle penetrating a hyperalgesic area may stimulate C fibres and cause more pain and distress to the patient. In these cases a perisegmental approach is recommended, i.e. needling either side of the affected segment or segments. In some cases needles may be placed even further away from the painful area at distant sites, with the hope of generating a heterosegmental effect, reducing central sensitisation and, with subsequent treatments, be able to needle more closely to the source of pain.

With these considerations in mind, the treatment of true neuropathic or disc-related pain carries a guarded prognosis. The best chance of success with these cases would be to use electroacupuncture (see: Chapter 11).

REFERENCES

1. Onda A, Murata Y, Rydevik B, Larsson K, Kikuchi S, Olmarker K. Immunoreactivity of brain-derived neurotrophic factor in rat dorsal root ganglion and spinal cord dorsal horn following exposure to herniated nucleus pulposus. *Neurosci Lett* 2003;352(1):49–52.

2. Simons DG, Travell JG, Simons PT. *Travell & Simons' Myofascial Pain & Dysfunction. The Trigger Point Manual. Volume 1. Upper Half of Body. 2.* Baltimore: Williams & Wilkins; 1999.

3. Travell JG, Simons DG. *Myofascial Pain & Dysfunction. The Trigger Point Manual. Volume 1. The Upper Extremities. 1.* Baltimore: Williams & Wilkins; 1983.

4. Melzack R, Stillwell DM, Fox EJ. Trigger points and acupuncture points for pain: correlations and implications. *Pain* 1977;3(1):3–23.

5. Froriep R. Ein Beitrag zur Pathologie und Therapie des Rheumatismus. *Weimar* 1843.

6. Virchow R. Ueber parenchymatösa Entzündung. *Arch Path Anat* 1852;4:261–79.

7. Helleday U. Om myitis chronica (rheumatica). Et bidrag till dess diagnostik och behandling. *Nord Med Arch* 1876;8:Art.8.

8. Schade H. Untersuchungen in der Erkältungstrage: III. Uber den Rheumatismus, insbesondereden Muskelrheumatismus (Myogelosis). *Müench Med Wochenschr* 1921;68:95–9.

9. Lange F, Eversbusch G. Die bedeutung der Muskelhärten für die allgemeine Praxis. *Müench Med Wochenschr* 1921;68:418–20.

10. Gowers WR. Lumbago: its lessons and analogues. *BMJ* 1904;1:117–21.

11. Kellgren JH. Observations on referred pain arising from muscle. *Clin Sci* 1938;3:175–90.

12. Good MG. Objective diagnosis and curability of nonarticular rheumatism. *Br J Phys Med* 1951;14:1–7.

13. Kelly M. The nature of fibrositis: 1. The myalgic lesion and its secondary effects: a reflex theory. *Ann Rheum Dis* 1945;5:1–7.

14. Travell J. Myofascial trigger points: clinical view. In: Bonica JJ, Albe-Fessard D, editors. *Advances in Pain Research and Therapy Vol. 1.* New York: Raven Press; 1976. pp. 919–26.

15. Jacobsen S, Bartels EM, Danneskiold-Samsoe B. Single cell morphology of muscle in patients with chronic muscle pain. *Scand J Rheumatol* 1991;20(5):336–43.

16. Gerwin RD. Neurobiology of the myofascial trigger point. *Baillieres Clin Rheumatol* 1994;8(4):747–62.

17. Hubbard DR, Berkoff GM. Myofascial trigger points show spontaneous needle EMG activity. *Spine* 1993;18(13):1803–7.

18. Durette MR, Rodriquez AA, Agre JC, Silverman JL. Needle electromyographic evaluation of patients with myofascial or fibromyalgic pain. *Am J Phys Med Rehabil* 1991;70(3):154–6.

19. Couppé C, Midttun A, Hilden J, Jørgensen U, Oxholm P, Fuglsang-Frederiksen A. Spontaneous needle electromyographic activity in myofascial trigger points in the infraspinatus muscle: a blinded assessment. *J Musculoskelet Pain* 2001;9(3):7–16.
20. McNulty WH, Gevirtz RN, Hubbard DR, Berkoff GM. Needle electromyographic evaluation of trigger point response to a psychological stressor. *Psychophysiology* 1994;31(3):313–6.
21. Hubbard DR, Berkoff GM. Myofascial trigger points show spontaneous needle EMG activity. *Spine* 1993;18(13):1803–7.
22. Hong CZ, Simons DG. Pathophysiologic and electrophysiologic mechanisms of myofascial trigger points. *Arch Phys Med Rehabil* 1998;79(7):863–72.
23. Filshie J, Cummings TM. Western medical acupuncture. In: Ernst E, White A, editors. *Acupuncture – A Scientific Appraisal.* Oxford: Butterworth Heinemann; 1999. pp. 31–59.
24. Sola AE, Rodenberger ML, Gettys BB. Incidence of hypersensitive areas in posterior shoulder muscles. *Am J Phys Med* 1955;3:585–90.
25. Gerwin RD. A study of 96 subjects examined both for fibromyalgia and myofascial pain. *J Musculoskelet Pain* 1995;3(Suppl 1):121.
26. Fishbain DA, Goldberg M, Meagher BR, Steele R, Rosomoff H. Male and female chronic pain patients categorized by DSM-III psychiatric diagnostic criteria. *Pain* 1986;26(2):181–97.
27. Fricton JR, Kroening R, Haley D, Siegert R. Myofascial pain syndrome of the head and neck: a review of clinical characteristics of 164 patients. *Oral Surg Oral Med Oral Pathol* 1985;60(6):615–23.
28. Skootsky SA, Jaeger B, Oye RK. Prevalence of myofascial pain in general internal medicine practice. *West J Med* 1989;151(2):157–60.
29. Chaiamnuay P, Darmawan J, Muirden KD, Assawatanabodee P. Epidemiology of rheumatic disease in rural Thailand: a WHO-ILAR COPCORD study. Community Oriented Programme for the Control of Rheumatic Disease. *J Rheumatol* 1998;25(7):1382–7.
30. Wolfe F, Simons DG, Fricton J, Bennett RM, Goldenberg DL, Gerwin R, Hathaway D, McCain GA, Russell IJ, Sanders HO. The fibromyalgia and myofascial pain syndromes: a preliminary study of tender points and trigger points in persons with fibromyalgia, myofascial pain syndrome and no disease. *J Rheumatol* 1992;19(6):944–51.
31. Jansenns LAA. Observations on acupuncture therapy in chronic osteoarthritis in dogs: A review of sixty one cases. *J Small Anim Pract* 1985;27(12):825–7.
32. Nice DA, Riddle DL, Lamb RL, Mayhew TP, Rucker K. Intertester reliability of judgments of the presence of trigger points in patients with low back pain. *Arch Phys Med Rehabil* 1992;73(10):893–8.
33. Njoo KH, Van der Does E. The occurrence and inter-rater reliability of myofascial trigger points in the quadratus lumborum and gluteus medius: a prospective study in non-specific low back pain patients and controls in general practice. *Pain* 1994;58(3):317–23.

34. Gerwin RD, Shannon S, Hong CZ, Hubbard D, Gevirtz R. Interrater reliability in myofascial trigger point examination. *Pain* 1997;69(1–2):65–73.

35. Cummings TM, White AR. Needling therapies in the management of myofascial trigger point pain: a systematic review. *Arch Phys Med Rehabil* 2001;82(7):986–92.

36. Garvey TA, Marks MR, Wiesel SW. A prospective, randomized, double-blind evaluation of trigger-point injection therapy for low-back pain. *Spine* 1989;14(9):962–4.

37. Hong CZ. Lidocaine injection versus dry needling to myofascial trigger point. The importance of the local twitch response. *Am J Phys Med Rehabil* 1994;73(4):256–63.

38. Cummings TM, White AR. Needling therapies in the management of myofascial trigger point pain: a systematic review. *Arch Phys Med Rehabil* 2001;82(7):986–92.

39. Lewit K. The needle effect in the relief of myofascial pain. *Pain* 1979;6(1):83–90.

40. Cummings TM. A computerised audit of acupuncture in two populations: Civilian and Forces. *Acupunct Med* 1996;14(1):37–9.

41. Sonkin LS. Therapeutic trials with thyroid hormones in chemically euthyroid patients with myofascial pain and complaints suggesting mild thyroid insufficiency. *J Back Musculoskeletal Rehabil* 1997;8(2):165–71.

42. Hong CZ, Simons DG. Pathophysiologic and electrophysiologic mechanisms of myofascial trigger points. *Arch Phys Med Rehabil* 1998;79(7):863–72.

43. Berman BM, Lao L, Langenberg P, Lee WL, Gilpin AM, Hochberg MC. Effectiveness of acupuncture as adjunctive therapy in osteoarthritis of the knee: a randomized, controlled trial. *Ann Intern Med* 2004;141(12):901–10.

44. Vas J, Mendez C, Perea-Milla E, Vega E, Panadero MD, Leon JM, Borge MA, Gaspar O, Sanchez-Rodriguez F, Aguilar I, Jurado R. Acupuncture as a complementary therapy to the pharmacological treatment of osteoarthritis of the knee: randomised controlled trial. *BMJ* 2004;329(7476):1216.

45. Witt C, Brinkhaus B, Jena S, Linde K, Streng A, Wagenpfeil S, Hummelsberger J, Walther HU, Melchart D, Willich SN. Acupuncture in patients with osteoarthritis of the knee: a randomised trial. *Lancet* 2005;366(9480):136–43.

46. Jin Z, Tao Z, Ren W, Du X. [Electro-acupuncture effects on experimental spinal cord injury of the cat as evaluated by acid phosphatase detection.] *Chen Tzu Yen Chiu* 1996;21(4):50–3.

47. Politis MJ, Korchinski MA. Beneficial effects of acupuncture treatment following experimental spinal cord injury: a behavioral, morphological, and biochemical study. *Acupunct Electrother Res* 1990;15(1):37–49.

48. Yang JW, Jeong SM, Seo KM, Nam TC. Effects of corticosteroid and electroacupuncture on experimental spinal cord injury in dogs. *J Vet Sci* 2003;4(1):97–101.

Principles of point selection 7

From a neurophysiological perspective, stimulation of A delta or type III fibres in the dorsal horn of the spinal segment of the painful area will maximise competition with C fibre ('slow') pain, thereby inhibiting it. This inhibition occurs mainly in layer II of the substantsia gelatinosa of the dorsal horn of the spinal cord. The inhibition created by stimulation of A delta fibres is necessarily limited by the possible area of inhibitory affect of the area of action of the fibre stimulated. In essence this means that the acupuncture needle should be inserted as close as possible to the source of pain. For musculoskeletal problems, this usually means putting the needle where it hurts.

In human patients, we can either ask them where it hurts or search for a distant trigger point that reproduces their pain. In animals, we cannot be completely sure where it hurts or that an area hurts at any time other than when we are palpating it, but there are some clues:

(1) Radiography, MRI scan or other imagining techniques may localise a lesion that we assume is painful because of its position, size, the degree of abnormality or destructive effect on adjacent tissues.
(2) Examination of joints may reveal: crepitus, restriction of movement, swelling, heat or bony distortion, all of which are assumed to accompany painful and active conditions such as osteoarthritis, although some could also indicate disc disease, tumour or neuropathic pain.
(3) Examination of muscles may reveal tender areas that one would not normally expect to be tender. If these are in the same muscle group as the diseased joint, for example, it may be assumed that this tenderness is a problem for the animal.

(4) Examination of the muscles may reveal myofascial trigger points. These trigger points may be in muscle groups associated with the diseased joint, or in the region of spinal abnormality, or in muscles that now bear the biomechanical strain of altered posture. So, for hip arthritis always check the lumbar and thoracic epaxial muscles and the muscles of the shoulder girdle. For a unilaterally painful joint or limb conditions always check the contralateral limb girdle. The distribution of pain and trigger points in animals with multiple problems can give a clue as to which limb bothers them most. Experience and the animal's response to palpation is the guide as to which of the trigger points are likely to be most active.

(5) Requesting information about movement could be helpful, for example: a dog may present with a diagnosis of hip arthritis and radiographically demonstrate some mild changes in the elbows, but the history reveals no difficulty in climbing stairs. The problem for the animal may be going *down* stairs. There is likely to be widespread tenderness on examination, but the patient may be *suffering* from the pain in its forequarters more significantly because it has to throw more of its weight forward.

(6) Regions of hyperalgesia (perceiving noxious stimuli is more painful than usual) and allodynia (perceiving non-noxious stimuli, such as light touch, as painful) are indicative of pain and central sensitisation in that area of the body. Classically there is muscle trembling and fasciculation on light touch, or sharp withdrawal of the limb when passing a hand near the affected region or body.

Having taken all these clues into account the principles are:

- Acupuncture active trigger points.
- Acupuncture relevant tender areas.
- Needle acupuncture points close to the painful area.

LOCAL NEEDLING

From a Western neurophysiological perspective, local needling is probably all that is needed, however the principles of distant needling are mentioned here for the sake of completeness. In traditional Chinese medicine much emphasis was placed on this concept. The idea is that adding a needle in a part of the body distant from the area being treated adds to the overall effect. There is no evidence to suggest that this is the case, although it would not be 'wrong' to practise this technique.

DISTANT NEEDLING

(1) Acupuncture points that are segmental for the diseased or painful area.
(2) Acupuncture points on the meridian that passes through the diseased or painful area.
(3) Needle acupuncture points distant from the site of the disease or pain that seem more tender than one would expect.

Principles

The principles of distant needling are illustrated here by the example of a simple, relatively short-lived condition, such as recent onset of pain and lameness from osteochondrosis dissecans in the shoulder of a six-month-old Labrador. Examination is likely to reveal pain on palpation of the joint, some tenderness in adjacent muscles and trigger points in infraspinatus and triceps muscles on the ipsilateral side. Local needling would be to the active trigger points in infraspinatus and triceps muscles, any especially tender areas adjacent to the joint and to the acupuncture point over the shoulder that is called LI15 (shown in Figure 7.1). This may be tender and therefore overlap two of the principles in consideration of its needling. The trigger point in infraspinatus may well coincide with the acupuncture point SI11 (shown in Figure 7.2) and would satisfy local needling principles on all three accounts. This is shown in Figure 7.3.

If one were then to choose distant points, the principles would suggest another point in the large intestine meridian, such as LI11 over the elbow, or LI4 near the dew claw (shown in Figure 7.1). The caudal trapezius muscle on the ipsilateral side may be tender and one could choose to needle the opposite limb to access the same spinal segment. In this case SI11 may well be tender (more weight on this side), is on a relevant meridian and is a segmental point and therefore would satisfy all three principles for the selection of distant points (shown in Figure 7.4).

Note that it is not necessary or even always possible to find the 'overlap'; this is just an illustration of the principles. In most patients the picture would be much more complicated and treatment of distant points would overlap with treatments of points that are local to other

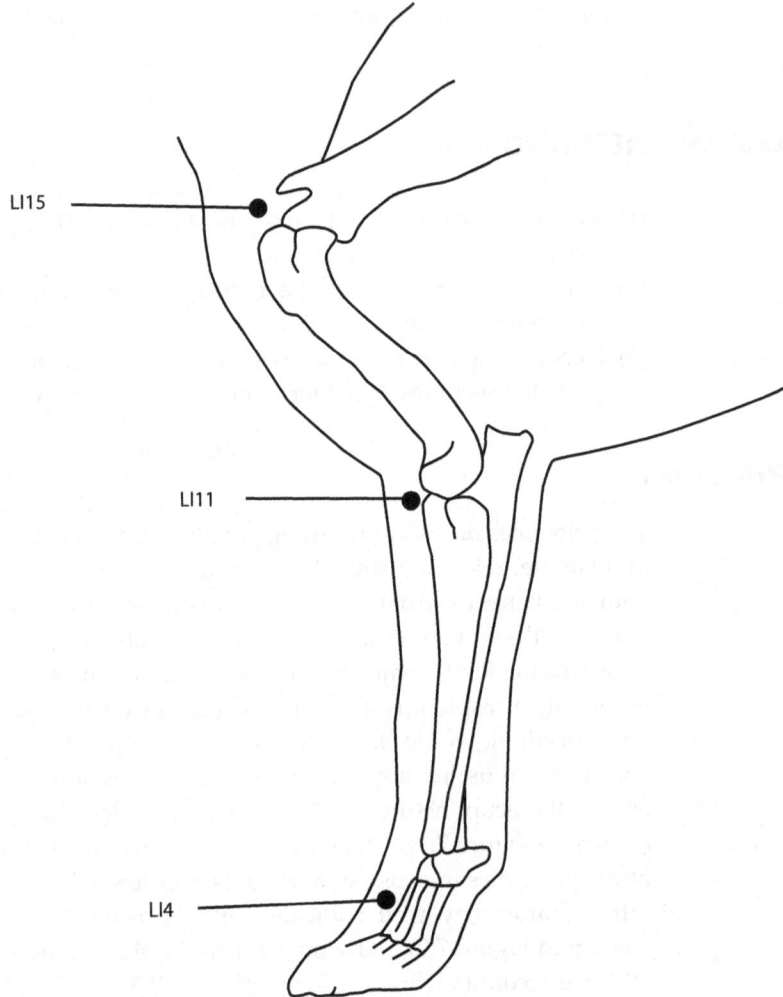

LI15

LI11

LI4

Figure 7.1 Position of LI4, LI11 and LI15 in the dog. LI4 in dogs is located between the dew claw and the second metacarpal bone. LI11 is found halfway between the lateral epicondyle of the humerus and the biceps tendon. LI15 is found in the depression at the cranial tip of the acromium.

problematic areas. In the example given, if the problem continued, then there may well be active trigger points on the contralateral limb, in caudal trapezius because of the tendency to lean backwards to take pressure off the affected limb, and even in epaxial muscles on the contralateral side for the same reason.

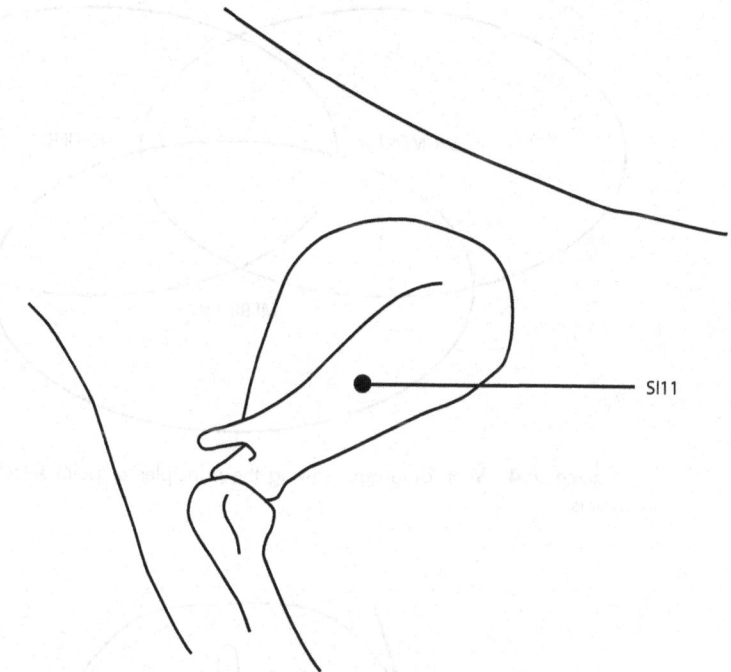

Figure 7.2 Position of SI11 or Small Intestine 11 in the infraspinatus muscle of the dog.

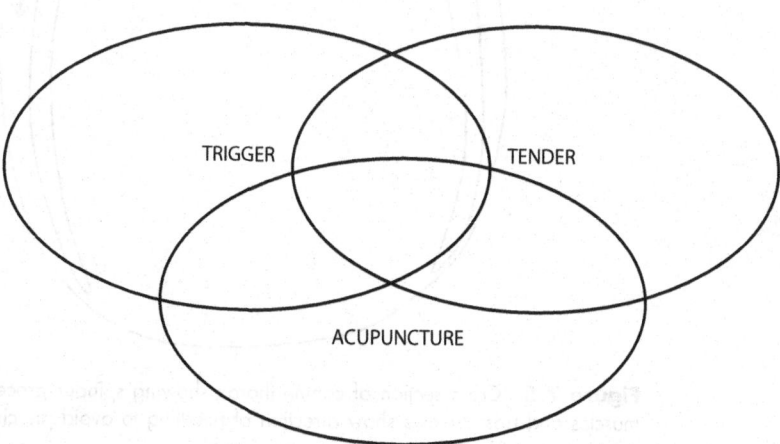

Figure 7.3 Venn diagram showing the principles of point selection for local points.

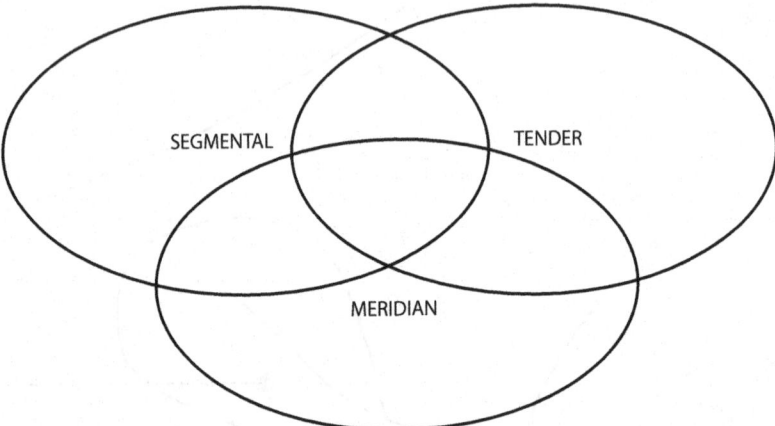

Figure 7.4 Venn diagram showing the principles of point selection for distant points.

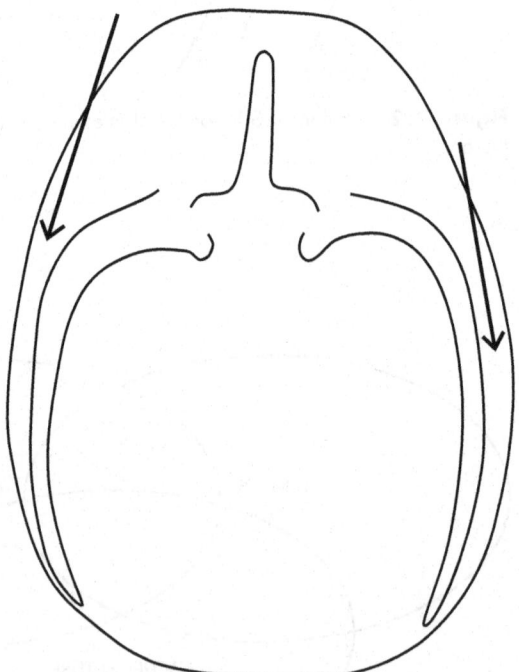

Figure 7.5 Cross section of canine thorax showing spinous process, epaxial muscles and ribs. Arrows show direction of needling to avoid piercing the pleura.

Remember that when one is treating a musculoskeletal problem, segmental acupuncture is practised anyway when the painful area is needled. Sticking the needle where it hurts equals segmental acupuncture, so most of the time there does not need to be a conscious decision about where to needle the relevant segment. This may become relevant if one is treating, for example, an apparent phantom limb pain (no local points!) or neuropathic pain (too painful to needle directly) or an oedematous limb (risk of infection). In these cases the opposite limb can be used, or paraspinal needling (see: Chapter 9).

Safety considerations (also see: Chapter 1)

(1) In needling over the thorax avoid needling between the ribs because of the risk of pneumothorax. To avoid this:

- Needle tangentially as shown in Figure 7.5
- Needle superficially
- Needle over a rib.

(2) Deep needling above the level of L4 in the midline in dogs and cats carries a theoretical risk of spinal cord damage or infection.

(3) Avoid needling into joint spaces.

(4) Care with immunocompromised patients.

(5) Care with needling patients with coagulopathies and bleeding disorders, especially when needling in closed fascial compartments, because of the risk of compartment syndrome.

(6) Avoid leaving needles in place where dogs can easily reach them. Labradors will assume anything novel is edible until proven otherwise. Needles left in distal forelimbs are fair game. Brief needling techniques in these areas may be safer.

Acupuncture for the treatment of visceral pain and dysfunction

8

SEGMENTAL ACUPUNCTURE

Definition:

The term segmental acupuncture is used to describe the technique of needling any structure innervated by the same spinal segment as the disordered structure under treatment.

When musculoskeletal problems are treated, they can usually be needled directly, for example: an arthritic stifle would be treated by needling points around the stifle as well as any associated myofascial trigger points. This is local needling. It is also segmental – where one stimulates the stifle directly, the spinal segment that innervates the stifle is being stimulated.

However, there may be circumstances in which direct, local needling is not possible, for example:

(1) The limb may have been amputated. In humans, phantom limb pain is a challenging and often refractory problem post amputation. It is not a phenomenon commonly discussed in veterinary medicine, but from a neurophysiological viewpoint there is no reason why animals should *not* experience sensations from the absent limb.

(2) More commonly, the stifle may not be accessible. For example: postoperatively one may want to avoid the operation site – the area may be hyperalgesic and simply too painful to needle, or the limb may be oedematous.

111

In these circumstances we need to find another part of the soma inner-vated by the same spinal segment that innervates (in this case) the stifle. Needling the opposite limb would be a possibility; higher on the same limb may be appropriate; or needling paraspinally at the appropriate level, which will be described later, should achieve a similar effect.

So far this is fairly straightforward, but problems potentially arise when the disordered, diseased or painful structure cannot be visu-alised or reached directly. Obviously, directly needling the gut or bladder is neither wise nor desirable, so the challenge is to find another structure innervated by the same spinal segment.

In order to achieve this it is important to have an understanding of the innervation of both the relevant visceral and somatic structures. In humans this is reasonably well documented and more fully under-stood than in animals. The most detailed equivalent knowledge has been described for the dog. Our knowledge of innervation in other species often seems to be dependent on its practical value in day-to-day veterinary medicine.

Illustration of the way in which our knowledge of innervation helps us to decide where to place acupuncture needles is best described in man. Detailed descriptions of dermatomes, myotomes and sclero-tomes are simply not available for most species and the information that is available comes from a variety of sources. Therefore, once the principles have been described in man, some general guidelines can be given on where to needle our non-human animal patients for vis-ceral conditions.

INNERVATION OF ABDOMINAL STRUCTURES IN MAN

The innervation of the abdominal wall is straightforward. There is a sequential pattern of afferent and efferent supply from the intercostal nerves: T7 at the epigastrium to T10 at the umbilicus and L1 at the level of the pubic symphysis. Visceral innervation is more complex and involves the autonomic nervous system.

The autonomic nervous system is the part of the nervous system concerned with the innervation of involuntary structures, such as the heart, smooth muscle and glands throughout the body. It is made up of sympathetic and parasympathetic components. The activities of the sympathetic part of the autonomic nervous system prepare the body for an emergency by redistributing blood from the skin and intestine to the brain, heart and skeletal muscle and by inhibiting peristalsis and closing the sphincters. The activities of the parasympathetic part of the autonomic nervous system aim at conserving and restoring energy. These slow the heart rate, increase intestinal peristalsis and glandular activity and open the sphincters.

> Note that, whilst acupuncture has effects on the autonomic nervous system, it is not possible to have a direct targeted effect on either the sympathetic or parasympathetic component by needling. Acupuncture has a **normalising effect** on the autonomic nervous system.

Sympathetic efferent fibres are derived from the lateral grey horns of the spinal cord between T1 and L2. These myelinated, preganglionic fibres leave the spinal cord via the ventral nerve roots and pass via the white rami communicantes to the paravertebral ganglia of the sympathetic trunk. Here they either synapse or continue to more distant ganglia. These ganglia may be higher or lower on the sympathetic chain, or associated with the branches of the abdominal aorta. Myelinated, preganglionic nerves originating from T5 to T9 pass through the ganglia of the sympathetic trunk to form the greater splanchnic nerve and the fibres go on to synapse in the ganglia of the coeliac plexus. The lesser splanchnic nerve arises in a similar fashion from T10 and T11 and its fibres proceed to the coeliac, superior mesenteric or aorticorenal ganglia. When present, the lowest splanchnic nerve arises from T12 and its fibres end in the aorticorenal ganglion.

Unmyelinated, postganglionic sympathetic efferents from the coeliac ganglion supply the stomach (T6 to T10) and other fibres pass via the superior mesenteric ganglion to supply the small intestine, ascending and transverse colon (T9 to L1). The distal third of the transverse colon, the descending colon and the pelvic viscera are supplied from L1 and L2 via four lumbar splanchnic nerves. The two superior lumbar splanchnic nerves end in the inferior mesenteric ganglion and the two inferior nerves join the superior hypogastric plexus.

The parasympathetic efferents originate in the nuclei of cranial nerves 3, 7, 9 and 10 and in the grey matter of the second, third and fourth sacral segments of the spinal cord. Most of the abdominal viscera are supplied via preganglionic parasympathetic fibres that run in the vagus nerves and synapse close to the viscera concerned. The distal third of the transverse colon, the descending colon and pelvic viscera derive their parasympathetic supply from S2, S3 and S4, via the pelvic splanchnic nerves and inferior hypogastric plexus.

It is important to remember that the afferent component of the autonomic nervous system is identical to that of somatic nerves. The nerve endings of the autonomic afferents are stimulated by stretch or chemical changes (e.g. those resulting from a lack of oxygen in the tissues) rather than heat or touch, but once the fibres gain entrance to the spinal cord they travel alongside, or are mixed with, the somatic afferent fibres.

Abdominal pain

Abdominal pain arising from the parietal peritoneum is of the somatic type and can be precisely localised. This pain is often severe in nature. The visceral peritoneum has no afferent pain fibres, but the root of the mesentery is very sensitive to stretch. The gastrointestinal tract arises embryologically as a midline structure and receives a bilateral nerve supply. Because of this origin, pain arising from an abdominal viscus is dull, poorly localised and referred to the midline, depending on segmental innervation. Pain from the stomach and duodenum is felt in the epigastrium; from the jejunum to the transverse colon in the umbilical region; and from the transverse colon to the rectum in the hypogastrium. These areas of pain referral are sometimes termed 'Head areas' or 'zones' after the English neurologist (Sir Henry Head), who described skin hypersensitivity over areas of pain referral from viscera.

Somatovisceral and viscerosomatic effects

There appears to be a relationship between somatic pathology and visceral symptoms (somatovisceral effects) and between visceral pathology and somatic symptoms (viscerosomatic effects). Simons, Travell and Simons describe diarrhoea, vomiting, food intolerance, colic and dysmenorrhoea resulting from trigger points in the abdominal wall musculature[1]. They also describe the activation of trigger points in the abdominal wall secondary to pain derived from visceral disease, such as a peptic ulcer. Such trigger points can cause persistence of symptoms despite resolution of the visceral pathology. But perhaps the most well recognised viscerosomatic effect is the rigid abdomen of a patient with peritonitis.

It is not surprising then that abdominal symptoms are often the source of diagnostic confusion. Consider the common presenting symptom of right iliac fossa pain in man. There are many possible sources of nociceptive pain that can be perceived in this area:

(1) Visceral sources of pain:
  • Appendicitis
  • Torsion, haemorrhage or rupture of a right ovarian cyst
  • Right salpingitis
  • Torsion of the right testicle
  • Inflammatory bowel disease with involvement of the terminal ileum.

(2) Somatic sources of pain:
  • Myofascial trigger point (TrP) in the right lower rectus abdominis
  • TrP in the right external oblique
  • TrP in the right iliocostalis thoracis (T11 level)
  • TrP in right multifidi (S1 level)
  • TrP high in right adductors
  • Right inguinal hernia
  • Irritation of nerve roots at T12 or L1
  • Degeneration of zygapophyseal joints on the right at T12 to L2.

Somatovisceral and viscerosomatic effects have not been described in the veterinary species, but there is no reason to suppose that they do not exist. One of the authors (SL) has found asymmetrical and painful trigger points in the abdominal wall of patients with low-grade and persistent gastrointestinal signs, but this can hardly be cited as proof of any causative factor. It would be valuable to investigate this further in a population of suitable patients.

APPROACH TO TREATMENT IN ANIMALS

In order to apply these principles of treatment to non-human animals it is necessary that we have at least a general understanding of the innervation of the viscera we hope to influence. There is incomplete knowledge of the path of the autonomic nervous system in the horse and the ruminant. It would be prudent, therefore, to treat several segments at the same time, and to treat paraspinal points, since with these we have some confidence about the level at which we are treating. Although points such as BL23 have been used traditionally to influence the bladder, and it has segmental relevance in humans, it cannot be concluded with confidence that this will be true in all species. BL23 and BL25 (Figure 8.1) are included in many formulae

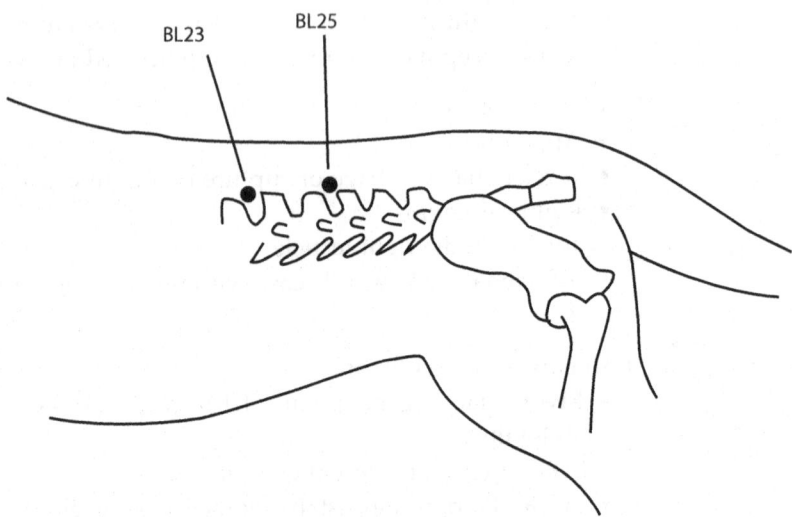

Figure 8.1 BL23 and BL25 in the dog. The points are in longissimus muscles.

for bladder and bowel disorders in animals, however, a segmental approach to treatment should focus on paraspinal points at the relevant levels.

Canine autonomic system

Some general effects of the autonomic system are known for the dog[2]. In terms of the sympathetic innervation, the cranial thoracic segments affect the iris and ciliary muscle of the eye, dilating the pupil and relaxing the muscle. The same segments stimulate vasoconstriction of the salivary glands and contraction of their myoepithelial cells, vasoconstriction of the lacrimal gland and increased activity of the heart. The thoracic and lumbar segments cause vasoconstriction of blood vessels in the skin and vasodilation of skeletal muscle vessels. The caudal thoracic segments stimulate relaxation of the bronchii and secretion from the adrenal medulla; the same segments along with the lumbar segments cause decreased activity in the intestinal tract. Finally, the lumbar segments cause relaxation of the bladder wall.

The parasympathetic innervation targets the iris and ciliary muscle via the oculomotor nerve causing pupil contraction and accommodation for near vision. The facial and glossopharyngeal nerves stimulate vasodilation and secretion in the salivary glands, while the facial nerve alone causes the lacrimal glands to secrete. The vagus stimulates reduced activity in the heart, vasodilation or vasoconstriction in blood vessels, depending on their site, and, along with the pelvic nerves, increases motility and secretion in the intestinal tract. The pelvic nerves stimulate contraction of the bladder wall and vasodilation of erectile tissue.

URINARY PROBLEMS

Canine bladder innervation

Reflex function of the canine bladder is mediated through sacral segments: pelvic parasympathetic nerves and the somatic pudendal nerve. Bladder function is also influenced by upper motor neuron pathways from the caudal brain stem, cerebellum and cerebrum.

Stretch and pressure receptors in the bladder wall relay via the pelvic nerves to sacral segments and complete a reflex arc via motor efferents as well as ascending to higher centres in the spinal cord and the brain.

Parasympathetic innervation arises from S1 to S3 in dogs and cats (S2–S4 in ruminants), acting on the bladder wall to contract the detrusor muscle and passively dilate the neck of the bladder.

Sympathetic innervation originates in L1 to L4 spinal cord segments in dogs and L2 to L5 in cats. This innervation acts upon the wall and neck of the bladder via splanchnic nerves and the caudal mesenteric ganglion.

In normal micturition, visceral afferent stimulation inhibits sympathetic and somatic pathways leading to a decrease in tone of the bladder neck, urethra and striated urinary sphincter. This stimulation also facilitates parasympathetic mediation of detrusor contraction.

Urinary incontinence

Post-spaying urinary incontinence is thought to be due to removal of the oestrogenic influence on the bladder sphincter (sphincter mechanism incompetence) and an increase in external pressure on the bladder secondary to a change in its position from the abdominal to the pelvic cavity.

Both conventional treatments (oestrogen replacement or sympathomimetic drugs) may have unacceptable side effects in some individuals. Acupuncture may be able to modulate visceral afferent activity and normalise bladder function. In humans the evidence is that acupuncture is as effective as the conventional treatment of oxy-butynin[3], an anticholinergic agent for detrusor instability, but this is not the same aetiology as canine urinary incontinence. However, if acupuncture could have an effect on canine bladder function, afferent activity is likely to be modulated most effectively by segmental acupuncture. As in humans, visceral afferents are likely to travel with both sympathetic and parasympathetic nerves, so paraspinal needling at L1 to L4 and at S1 to S3 would appear to be a reasonable option for acupuncture treatment.

The best evidence in animals that we have for this is from Sato *et al.* who demonstrated that an effect of acupuncture in reducing spontaneous bladder contraction in rats only occurs with segmental needling[4].

In practice, the results appear to be mixed, with some practitioners claiming good results, others equivocal and some completely negative. It is possible that the stimulation has not been robust enough, or that the needles have not been inserted deeply enough in the relevant muscles to affect the correct segmental level. Traditionally the Bladder points, which run parallel to the spine, as shown in Figure 8.2, in two lines (the inner and outer Bladder meridian), have been used to treat these kinds of problems. While this sounds logical and rather neat, it is possible that needling at this point into longissimus muscles may be stimulating segments at a level higher than L1 because of the way that long muscles drag their innervation during embryological development. In other words, needling superficial epaxial muscles adjacent to L1 to L4 is not likely to stimulate spinal segments L1 to L4. It is more likely that the innervation of these muscles is by the lower thoracic segments. Needling at these points is therefore only likely to

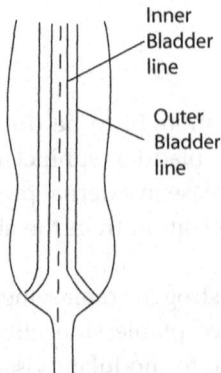

Inner
Bladder
line

Outer
Bladder
line

Figure 8.2 The Bladder meridians are traditionally said to run in two lines parallel to the spine – the inner and outer Bladder line. Paraspinal needling occurs inside the inner Bladder line, close to the spine.

have comparatively weak heterosegmental effects and the evidence (Sato *et al.*) is that segmental effects are needed[4].

In practice, we get around this difficulty by paraspinal needling (closer to the midline than the inner Bladder line) so that we can be relatively certain of the level at which we are stimulating.

Other causes of negative results in practice could be: that not enough cases have been attempted; that only challenging cases are tried as a last resort; that there have been other pathological factors influencing bladder function; that the stimulation has not been robust or frequent enough; or that owners have not persisted long enough with the treatment.

The other possibility is that, of course, acupuncture may not be an appropriate intervention for this problem or that it may only work in a small section of the affected population. Logically it would seem sensible to try acupuncture in that subsection of cases that has responded to the sympathomimetic agents. If the patient is experiencing unacceptable side effects with medication then there is little to lose, although the prognosis for response based on current field information should be guarded.

Urinary retention

Efficacy of treatment may depend upon whether the dysfunction is caused by upper motor neuron disease or lower motor neuron disease. Treatment of lower motor neuron bladder problems carries a better prognosis with conventional therapy, but probably also with acupuncture, which may act to facilitate parasympathetic stimulation of the detrusor muscle, as well as affecting somatic and sympathetic efferents, via modulation of segmental afferent activity.

These cases are always more urgent than incontinence problems and must carry a guarded prognosis. There is no strong evidence to suggest effectiveness either way, but it would be prudent to recommend relatively frequent (every few days) and relatively robust (probably electroacupuncture if tolerated) treatment.

GASTROINTESTINAL DISEASE

The same principles apply when considering gastrointestinal disease in the veterinary species. Sympathetic fibres arising from caudal thoracic segments supply the upper part of the gastrointestinal tract and the large intestine and rectum is supplied from caudal thoracic and lumbar segments. The parasympathetic supply comes from both the vagus and the pelvic nerves, the latter arising from sacral segments of the spinal cord. As a general rule, sympathetic efferent fibres decrease activity in the GI tract, and parasympathetic fibres increase motility and secretion, but remember that with acupuncture the effect is to **normalise function**, not to tweak one or other part of the autonomic system as is thought appropriate for the condition. Background activity is probably generated from the enteric nervous system, which runs within the wall of the GI tract and throughout its length.

Guidelines

Whether one is attempting to treat diarrhoea or constipation there are some clear guidelines to observe:

(1) Pathological causes of gastrointestinal disturbance should be ruled out as far as possible, including the use of strict exclusion diet, before using acupuncture to attempt to normalise the function of the gut. In all cases a diagnosis should be made as far as is possible to do so. Acupuncture can be a potent analgesic and it is possible that it could mask a serious underlying problem.

(2) Conditions with an obvious obstruction or lesion present are unlikely to be amenable to treatment with acupuncture.

(3) Acupuncture can modulate the afferent signals from the gastrointestinal tract; however, the subsequent effect on sympathetic and parasympathetic efferent nerves is likely to depend on the background activity in these systems. Experimental work seems to support the idea that somatic stimulation (acupuncture) has a normalising effect on autonomic tone, rather than consistently causing a change in one or other direction[5].

CONDITIONS TREATED

Gastrointestinal disease

Conditions such as irritable bowel syndrome (and there is still controversy about such a diagnosis in the veterinary species), when all other causes have been ruled out, would be the kind of *functional* problem that may be considered appropriate for treatment with acupuncture.

Megacolon and other functional causes of constipation in cats appear to be particularly susceptible to treatment with acupuncture, based on a small number of cases. Whether this is because cats may be especially sensitive generally to acupuncture, whether the aetiology of this condition lends itself to this kind of treatment or whether the non-specific effects of intervention are particularly potent, is unknown.

Ileus in rabbits and horses where normal function is possible, but disrupted, should be amenable to treatment but no information is available as to effectiveness.

Reproductive medicine

Acupuncture is used in an attempt to treat fertility problems in humans, however, there is little evidence to support this practice to date. Work in Sweden has demonstrated a change in uterine artery impedance with segmental electroacupuncture that could be consistent with improved fertility[6]. It is reasonable to propose that somatic stimulation may influence functional abnormalities, however, it is unlikely that such stimulation could increase fertility above normal levels.

Acupuncture is commonly used to treat dysmenorrhoea in humans, but this condition is not recognised in other animals. Anecdotal reports describe vaginal and uterine prolapse in cattle and sheep successfully treated with acupuncture, but treatment time can be prolonged (20 minutes plus with electroacupuncture). Extradural lidocaine is cheap, rapidly effective, and associated with minimal risk. It is suggested therefore that it should be considered to be superior on welfare grounds.

There are reports of the use of acupuncture to improve fertility in cattle, but none at the level of randomised controlled trial.

APPROACH TO TREATMENT

Principles of segmental acupuncture

As has been illustrated so far, acupuncture is a form of somatic stimulation with either a direct effect on myofascial trigger points or an indirect effect mediated via the nervous system. In this section we are dealing with primary visceral pathology and this may only be treated *indirectly*.

Although treating the abdominal wall over the zone of pain referral from a visceral source (a guarded abdomen secondary to peritonitis for example) *sounds* local, it is not local treatment because the visceral afferents travel in the splanchnic nerves and the needling sensation is transmitted in somatic nerves.

So the signs of visceral disease may be treated by deactivating secondary trigger points and by indirect segmental stimulation. As abdominal and pelvic visceral afferents arise from T5 to L2, and from S2 to S4, there are a few points on the lower limb that overlap in segmental innervation. Interestingly, needling SP6, perhaps the most commonly used point for gynaecological and urological disorders in humans, would produce stimulation of S1 and S2 segments and thus overlap with the afferent supply to the uterus and urinary bladder. However, in animals, the point SP6 is located in an area where there is often little muscle or soft tissue in which to insert the needle (Figure 8.3) and needling here is more awkward and likely to be resented by some patients. Therefore, while it may be a convenient site to access S1 and S2 segments in humans it is of less relevance in the veterinary species (from a neurophysiological perspective) and veterinarians have easy access to sacral segments by needling directly over the sacrum (acupuncture point BL28 for example) (Figure 8.4).

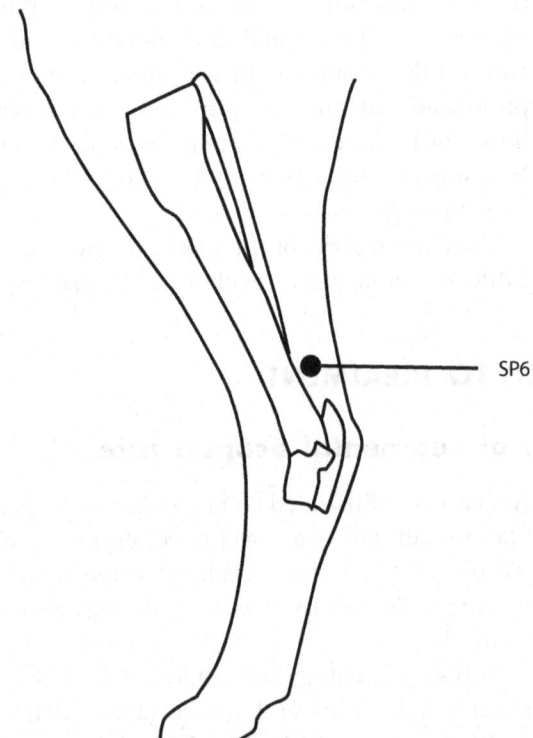

SP6

Figure 8.3 SP6 is located about one fifth of the way up the medial aspect of the tibia between the tibia and peroneus longus and flexor hallucis longus muscles.

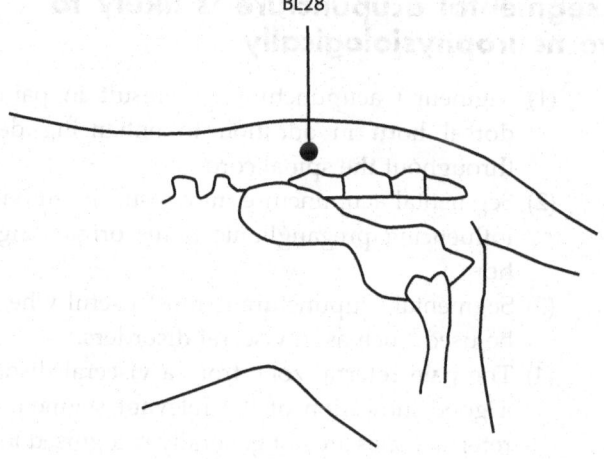

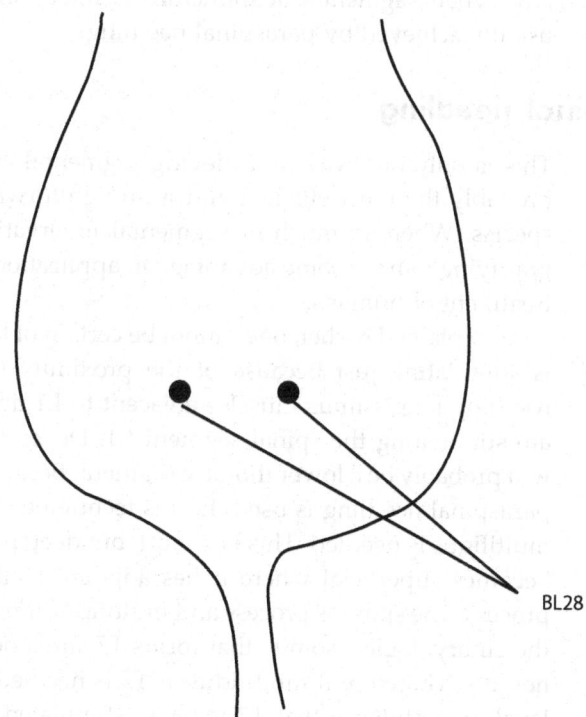

Figure 8.4 BL28 is located in the muscles over the sacrum; the diagrams show lateral and dorsal view.

What segmental acupuncture is likely to achieve neurophysiologically

(1) Segmental acupuncture will result in pain modulation at the dorsal horn in addition to enhancing descending inhibition throughout the spinal cord.

(2) Segmental acupuncture may result in autonomic modulation by influencing preganglionic fibres originating in the lateral grey horn.

(3) Segmental acupuncture is most useful when local points cannot be used, such as in visceral disorders.

(4) The pain referral zone from a visceral disorder is likely to give a good indication of the relevant segment to treat. While pain referral zones are not generally recognised in animals, for visceral disorders these are indicated from the response to clinical examination.

NB: When segmental acupuncture is intentionally performed it is usually achieved by paraspinal needling.

Paraspinal needling

This is only one way of achieving segmental acupuncture, but it is probably the most efficient and is straightforward in the veterinary species. When so much of segmental innervation is uncertain it is gratifying to have some advantage in application of this method over treatment of humans.

As explained earlier, one cannot be certain of the level at which one is stimulating just because of the proximity of the vertebrae, i.e. needling longissimus muscles adjacent to L1 does not mean that we are stimulating the spinal segment L1. Depending on the species it will probably be a lower thoracic segment. Because of this uncertainty, paraspinal needling is used. In this technique the paraspinal muscle multifidus is needled. This is a short, but deep paraspinal muscle that becomes superficial where it lies adjacent to the vertebral spinous process. The spinous process and multifidus muscle, which arise from the embryological somite that forms T7, are innervated by the spinal nerve 7. Therefore if multifidus at T7 is needled there can be a good level of confidence that T7 is being stimulated. All other structures innervated by T7 may then be affected by the competition at the dorsal horn at T7.

If the required levels for a bladder problem are L1 to L4 and S1 to S2 in the dog, then needling of multifidus muscles should occur bilaterally at at least two, if not three, sites between L1 and L4 and over the sacrum at BL28 which is, in effect, the multifidus for the sacral segments.

Practicalities of paraspinal needling

The safest technique is to needle at 45° between the spinous process and the lateral processes into muscle. This is shown in Figure 8.5. In humans the measurement from the midline of the spinous process is relatively consistent and is one fingerbreadth. Clearly this could not be a reliable measure in the veterinary species, even within one species, but it is a starting point and the advantage for the veterinary acupuncturist is that the spinous processes are much more prominent in our patients. Needling at this angle towards the spinous process ensures safety and access to multifidus at a more superficial level than if it is needled parallel to the spinous process.

Needling should occur bilaterally at each chosen segment and three or four segments from each range should be chosen to allow for errors in selecting level and for individual anatomical variation.

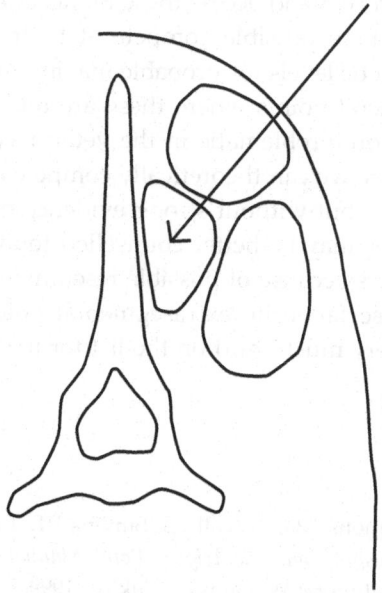

Figure 8.5 Paraspinal needling at 45° towards the spinous process through the epaxial muscles to multifidus muscles.

THE RELEVANCE OF TRADITIONAL APPROACHES

Study of traditional practice indicates frequent use of points that are clearly not segmental. It is well recognised that extrasegmental acupuncture stimulation can promote general analgesia and may have several other effects. Fortunately, there is some evidence that such stimulation can also affect visceral function, despite the evidence of Sato *et al.*[4,5] cited earlier. Tougas *et al.* demonstrated a reduction in basal gastric acid secretion with electroacupuncture in a series of controlled studies[7]. ST36 was used in the active group, which would not have directly stimulated T5 to T8, or the vagus, from which the autonomic innervation of the stomach is derived. In other words it is possible that one could have an effect wherever one needled – a rather annoying, but at the same time comforting, conclusion.

SUMMARY OF THE PRINCIPLES OF TREATMENT OF VISCERAL DISORDERS

(1) Treat any relevant trigger points in the abdominal wall or in the musculature of the back.
(2) Decide on the likely segments involved in the pathological process and access these by needling paraspinally.
(3) Where possible compete at both sympathetic and parasympathetic levels for probable maximum effect. In other words use the sacral points where these are relevant. Stimulating the vagus is more problematic in the veterinary species. In human acupuncture we can theoretically compete at this level by stimulating the ear, but without strong evidence of improved effects, veterinarians may be better counselled to avoid strong stimulation of the ears because of possible resentment by their patients.
(4) Use favourite extrasegmental points if tolerated (but these are very much third on the list for likely effect).

REFERENCES

1. Simons DG, Travell JG, Simons PT. *Travell & Simons' Myofascial Pain & Dysfunction. The Trigger Point Manual. Volume 1. Upper Half of Body.* 2. Baltimore: Williams & Wilkins; 1999.
2. Sack W, Wensing CJG, Dyce KM. *Textbook of Veterinary Anatomy.* Philadelphia: WB Saunders; 2002.

3. Kelleher CJ, Filshie J, Burton G, Khullar V, Cardozo ID. Acupuncture and the treatment of irritative bladder symptoms. *Acupunct Med* 1994;12(1):9–12.
4. Sato A, Sato Y, Suzuki A. Mechanism of the reflex inhibition of micturition contractions of the urinary bladder elicited by acupuncture-like stimulation in anesthetized rats. *Neurosci Res* 1992;15(3):189–98.
5. Sato A, Sato Y, Suzuki A, Uchida S. Neural mechanisms of the reflex inhibition and excitation of gastric motility elicited by acupuncture-like stimulation in anesthetized rats. *Neurosci Res* 1993;18(1):53–62.
6. Stener-Victorin E, Waldenstrom U, Andersson SA, Wikland M. Reduction of blood flow impedance in the uterine arteries of infertile women with electro-acupuncture. *Hum Reprod* 1996;11(6):1314–7.
7. Tougas G, Yuan LY, Radamaker JW, Chiverton SG, Hunt RH. Effect of acupuncture on gastric acid secretion in healthy male volunteers. *Dig Dis Sci* 1992;37(10):1576–82.

Acupuncture for the treatment of non-painful conditions

So far this text has mainly described acupuncture for painful, or potentially painful, conditions. This section includes a miscellany of conditions that are not necessarily regarded as primarily painful. However, the first to be considered are dermatological conditions, which may be painful and have some features in common with pain that bear discussion.

DERMATOLOGICAL CONDITIONS

Dermatological problems in companion animal practice account for a significant number of consultations. They can be frustrating, time-consuming, expensive for the owner and certainly a source of distress for the patient.

The integument

The skin can reflect underlying disease processes, e.g. hepatocutaneous syndrome, as well as succumbing to overwhelming stimuli from the environment, e.g. hypersensitivities to everything from dust mites to washing powder. Diagnosis is complicated by the fact that many lesions have become secondarily infected by the time they are presented to the practitioner.

The skin's function is protective and homeostatic as well as having other more specialised functions in certain species (e.g. camouflage; colour changes in reptiles).

129

The skin's simplest, hairless form is found at natural body orifices and on the feet of all species. Here it consists of an outer epidermis and an inner dermis consisting mainly of collagen and containing the deeper parts of glands that pass through the epidermis and open onto the skin surface. The dermoepidermal junction consists of papillae that attach the dermis to the epidermis and provide epidermal vascularisation. Most of the sensory nerve endings terminate here. The living dermis consists of keratinocytes, melanocytes, Langerhans cells and some other undefined cells. The keratinocytes move towards the surface, die, lose their nucleus, and form the horny outer layer of the epidermis.

The hairy integument differs from the above in that there is a relatively thin epidermis with less cornification, the presence of hairs and their associated structures, a dermoepidermal junction not usually formed into ridges and papillae and a greater mobility due to a looser attachment to underlying tissues.

At the digital extremities of mammals the epidermis produces a horny layer of much greater thickness and hardness than found in hairy skin. While this is related to friction at the surface, the effect is mediated via the dermis, e.g. the carnivore claw, the ungulate hoof, the chestnuts and ergots of the horse. The horns of ruminants also reflect a specialised adaptation of the integument.

Hairs develop from the epidermis. General body hairs are protective (e.g. against thermal changes) and are responsive to movement. Many species have both the larger guard hairs (present in all species) and an under fur (dog, cat and goat). Hair sheds and grows under the influence of temperature, nutrition, light intensity and duration, and disease.

Skin glands basically consist of sebaceous glands and sweat glands. Sebaceous glands arise as outgrowths from hair follicles. They produce sebum, which provides a protective coating, promotes dispersal of sweat across the skin, and provides a vehicle for pheromones. Sebaceous glands are influenced by the sex hormones.

Eccrine glands are the common sweat glands of the human skin. They occur over most of the body surface, except the axillae and anogenital region where apocrine glands occur. Eccrine glands are rare in domestic mammals, only being found in special sites such as the footpads of the dog and rodent, the carpal gland and muzzle of the pig and the muzzle of ruminants.

Apocrine glands are the major sweat gland in domestic animals. They are usually associated with primary hair follicles, although in some areas they open onto the skin surface. All species, except the pig, use sweat for evaporative cooling. The cat has poorly developed apocrine glands and relies on eccrine glands on the foot for cooling. The dog relies on footpad glands as well, but also has well developed dorsal apocrine glands. Ruminants sweat to lose body heat and the horse sweats profusely.

Acupuncture for dermatological problems

When treating dermatological conditions of the veterinary species the clinician has a number of general aims:

(1) To identify, if possible, the cause of the condition. Symptomatic treatment of dermatological problems with acupuncture should be used with caution where delay in diagnosis, masking of a serious underlying condition, or failure to identify a condition that renders acupuncture potentially more harmful (such as immunosuppression) could have serious consequences.

(2) To treat secondarily infected skin. Acupuncture is not a substitute for antibiotics where deep pyoderma is present, although it may be used adjunctively in wound healing.

(3) To reduce or eliminate pruritus. Itch undoubtedly causes suffering, self-trauma, more discomfort and continued distress. Animals may show adverse changes in behaviour because of significant skin problems, usually in terms of mood changes such as aggression or depression. Itch is transmitted along C fibres, ostensibly the same fibres that transmit slow pain. It has therefore long been thought that itch is a sort of sub-threshold pain and that itch can be transformed to pain by continued, more intense stimulation of the same C fibres. Using the same argument it has been postulated that, if acupuncture can compete with C fibre pain at the dorsal horn, thereby effectively blocking its onward transmission, then acupuncture should also be able to block the transmission of C fibre itch, thereby reducing pruritus. But here's the rub: dermatologists are currently in broad agreement (although this has changed in the past and may change again) that in fact itch is transmitted along *different* C fibres from those that transmit pain[1,2]. Since acupuncture appears not to be as effective for itch as one might suppose if it were competing with the C fibres in the same way as described for pain, this may help to explain why veterinary acupuncture practitioners do not, on the whole, get excited about the use of needling in the refractory atopic patient. However, there are some indications that acupuncture could be

useful in certain, sensitive individuals. There is also the influence of endorphins to consider: opiate peptides and their receptors in the CNS are involved in the perception of itch. Naloxone reduces the sensation of itch. Exogenous opiates relieve pain but exacerbate pruritus.

(4) To affect, where appropriate, the immune system, e.g. by the use of autogenous vaccines and by trying to eliminate the number of potential allergens in the environment or diet. Acupuncture appears to have an effect on the immune system, probably via endorphins, in much the same way that we know exercise can positively enhance it. These effects are not dramatic and are not going to rescue a severely compromised or abnormal immune system as far as it has been ascertained, but may normalise response in a sensitive individual.

(5) To establish and maintain skin hygiene.

There is some help from the literature to guide the practitioner to the kinds of dermatological conditions that may be useful to try treating:

Pruritus

When generalised, pruritus has many causes:

- Infestation
- Inflammation
- Neoplastic
- Metabolic
- Drug induced
- Idiopathic

Clearly it is important to make a diagnosis before trying acupuncture to suppress this complaint. It is of interest that no medication has ever been produced that will control itching satisfactorily.

A randomised controlled trial by Belgrade et al. in 1984[3] and a controlled trial by Lundeberg et al.[4] suggest that acupuncture is an effective inhibitor of histamine induced itch and flare, particularly when needling is applied in the same segment as the experimentally induced itch. This would suggest that acupuncture may be useful in conditions whose primary aetiology is histamine release, such as urticarial conditions, or perhaps those animals who have already responded positively to one of the many antihistamine preparations. The limitations of the information from these trials are:

- That the work was done on humans
- That the itch was experimentally induced in healthy individuals by an injection of histamine (therefore not reproducing the histamine release in a challenged and susceptible individual)
- That histamine is by no means the be all and end all of itch – if it were, one would expect more antihistamine preparations to be more effective more often

For the treatment of pathological pruritus, the human evidence is small and the veterinary evidence non-existent. In 1987 Duo showed an improvement in a small number ($n = 6$) of patients with uraemic pruritus who were treated with electrical nerve stimulation, a technique that in this case used needles[5]. A few small case series claimed a significant and long-lasting improvement in both uraemic pruritus and pruritus vulvae.

Because any anti-pruritic effect is likely to be generalised, the Western veterinary approach may justifiably choose any convenient, intramuscular points at which strong needling sensation can be produced. If pruritus is restricted to, or more prominent in, certain areas or segments, it would be logical to directly simulate those areas.

Wound healing

In the treatment of wounds healing by secondary intention, to speed up the healing of acral lick lesions (see later in this section) and to improve the healing of localised lesions, there is good indirect evidence from the literature that acupuncture is likely to be helpful.

In 1988 Lundeberg *et al.* demonstrated a significant improvement in objective measures of healing of ischaemic skin flaps in women who had undergone mastectomy[6]. In this case the treatment was electrical nerve stimulation (ENS) delivered via pads and not by needle penetration. This kind of stimulation may be considered to be more potent than dry needling, but not as potent as electroacupuncture. The treated women had significantly higher blood flow in the skin flaps and less evidence of oedema and stasis than those treated with a plausible placebo. This randomised controlled trial also demonstrated that those women who had normal blood flow in skin flaps at the start of the treatment did not have their blood flow altered, demonstrating once again the normalising effect of acupuncture and acupuncture-like stimuli.

A controlled experimental trial by Jansen *et al.* in 1989 looked at the healing of musculocutaneous skin flaps in rats and demonstrated that acupuncture significantly increased the likelihood of flap survival compared with controls; but that the needling had to be of sufficient depth into the tissue that one wanted to affect, and that the stimulus needed to be potent enough. In other words, superficial needling (just inserting the needle subcutaneously) and not stimulating it either manually or electrically did not increase flap survival[7]. Further work by Jansen *et al.*, 1989, in rats showed that the cause of the improved blood flow responsible for flap survival was an increase in local neurotransmitters[8]. These neurotransmitters, substance P and calcitonin gene-related peptide (CGRP), are potent vasodilators. Other neurotransmitters are released locally when acupuncture needles are inserted. Vasoactive intestinal peptide (VIP), another vasodilator, has been implicated in the healing of leg ulcers in man[9]; nerve growth factor stimulates the regrowth of local nerves into the wound[10], but also stimulates the release of other factors, and insulin growth factor has yet to have a clearly demonstrated role.

When an afferent nerve is stimulated, most of its neurotransmitters are released at the peripheral end of the nerve as described above. In a clinical setting an injury will stimulate the nerves and the release of neurotransmitters to accelerate healing and cause local sensitisation of the area to encourage guarding and protection. In acupuncture, stimulation of afferent nerves will release the neurotransmitters to encourage and accelerate healing and repair, but without the gross trauma and pain of injury.

The sum of the evidence available suggests that healing by secondary intention can be promoted by needling normal tissue around the circumference of the lesion, close to its margin. This technique is sometimes called 'Surrounding' or 'Fencing the Dragon'. General points to stimulate the immune system can also be used.

Acral lick dermatitis

Acral lick dermatitis is reported to be the most common canine psychodermatosis[11]. The cranial carpal and metacarpal areas are most commonly affected, but lesions may also be seen over the tarsus or metatarsus. Constant licking produces alopecia, followed by erosion and ulceration of the epidermis, often with subsequent secondary infections. The end result is a firm, raised, ulcerated plaque with a hyperpigmented halo. It is thought that the constant licking causes the production and release of endorphins, which have analgesic and euphoric effects to which the animal may become addicted. (Compulsive disorders are far more complicated than this and involve a multitude of neurotransmitters at different stages.)

Acral lick dermatitis may be purely of psychogenic origin but there can be underlying organic causes including hypersensitivities, hypothyroidism, bacterial and fungal diseases, foreign body reactions and underlying musculoskeletal pain[12,13]. Having excluded the possible organic causes, a thorough behavioural work-up is needed to identify sources of conflict or any underlying psychological cause.

Two acupuncture approaches have been described to treat this condition. The first is the insertion of needles into normal skin close to the margin of the lesion as described above ('Fencing the Dragon'), but many practitioners favour the second approach in which more general points are used, aimed at promoting healing by stimulation of the immune system and reducing pruritus. Anecdotally, owners of dogs treated successfully for this condition report a dramatic reduction in the compulsive nature of the licking. This may be due to a reduction in pruritus, enhanced wound healing, or indeed an effect on the compulsive behaviour mediated by alterations in serotonin or noradrenaline.

Other compulsive behaviours affecting the skin, such as excessive fur pulling and compulsive biting or licking of specific areas in cats, have also been responsive to acupuncture in anecdotal reports, but no formal studies have substantiated these suggestions.

Acral lick dermatoses are a challenge to treat in practice and, although it cannot be said with confidence that acupuncture is useful, it is likely to have an influence on at least some of the underlying causes. It is therefore probably worth trying after a thorough work-up and control of any deep pyoderma.

Summary of approach to dermatological conditions

Where there is an established and effective treatment for a specific condition this should be used first. Acupuncture can be used as an adjunctive therapy as part of a planned treatment.

For pruritus

(1) The Western approach would justify choosing any convenient intramuscular points at which strong needling sensation can be produced. If the pruritus is restricted to, or more prominent in, certain areas or segments, it would be logical to direct stimulation to those areas.
(2) Use local and surrounding points for distinct lesions.
(3) Use general points for widespread conditions.

(4) Conditions associated with primary histamine release may be more likely to respond.
(5) Consider underlying disease.

For wound healing

(1) Insert needles in healthy skin.
(2) Insert needles at the base of the flap or to surround the ulcerated area.
(3) For best results use high intensity electroacupuncture.
(4) Use repeated treatments once or twice a week.

For compulsive licking

(1) Use strong general points for maximal effects on behavioural neurotransmitters.
(2) Treat local lesions locally.
(3) Address possible spinal pain in cats overgrooming over lumbar spine.

EPILEPSY

A seizure can be defined as a transient clinical manifestation occurring as a result of a paroxysm of excessive electrical discharge within the brain. Seizures manifest as alterations in consciousness with or without motor activity and autonomic signs.

Epilepsy can be defined as recurrent seizure activity as a consequence of a brain dysfunction that is not associated with overt pathology; it may be congenital or acquired. Refractory epilepsy is seizure activity for which no primary cause can be found and for which appropriate anticonvulsant therapy has been given to no or insufficient effect.

In 1993 an article appeared in *Progress in Veterinary Neurology* by Luc Janssens[14] describing a case series of eleven dogs with epilepsy treated by ear acupuncture. His conclusions were that five of the eleven dogs showed that ear acupuncture may afford partial or complete seizure remission. In 1994 Panzer and Chrisman treated five dogs with refractory epilepsy by auricular acupuncture[15]. This case series reported a reduction in seizure activity in three dogs, one did not improve and one partially improved.

In both of these case series an attempt has been made to maintain the stimulation effects by inserting either small stay needles in the ears or gold implants (used because they are inert and should not cause a foreign body reaction at the site) at the site of acupuncture points.

Ear acupuncture has some practical and safety limitations and the evidence for its use probably does not justify its application over ordinary needling. The use of gold implants to maintain a stimulation effect could be argued to be self-defeating since constant stimulation at the same site may lead to an accommodation effect whereby the nerves no longer respond to the same repeated stimulus.

However, some veterinarians practising acupuncture report apparently good results when treating epilepsy, although the treatments need to be protracted. The problem with dealing with this kind of condition is the same as with any chronic disease in that it tends to change over time, its severity waxes and wanes and any positive improvement will be attributed to a novel intervention. To counter the anecdotal reports on the positive side, one of the authors (SL) observed a change after treating an epileptic Dalmation from having three or four seizures a month, to clustering the same number of seizures in one day. The owners were pleased because they felt this was easier to manage – the clinician did not agree and stopped the treatment! There have also been three cases of dogs with low-grade seizure activity receiving acupuncture for musculoskeletal disorders who have consistently seizured the day after treatment; their treatment was also suspended. There may be many potential non-specific effects of treatment and the events surrounding treatment that may trigger or suppress epilepsy; probably all these reports tend to indicate is that one has little chance of specifically affecting seizures in either direction, but obviously more controlled work would need to be done to establish this. A group of experienced veterinary acupuncturists meeting at the ABVA scientific study day in 2003 came to an almost unanimous consensus that they had little success in treating canine epilepsy by either a Western or traditional approach. One of the authors (SL) has been involved in some work looking at the role of diet in refractory epilepsy and it is clear that the long time frames involved and the elusive nature of the disease make assessing the outcome of any intervention problematic.

Summary

(1) There is no evidence above the level of case series that acupuncture works for refractory epilepsy.

(2) All efforts should be made to rule out any organic causes of seizures before concluding that the animal is suffering from idiopathic epilepsy.

(3) Anticonvulsant therapy should be maintained.

(4) An accurate diary of seizures should be kept.

(5) Points used are probably non-specific since the effects, if there are any, are likely to be generalised.

(6) It is worth warning owners that their epileptic pets may suffer seizures after acupuncture treatment. This warning is given to help avoid blame and litigation; not because there is any strong evidence that acupuncture can specifically cause a seizure. Some animals become exceptionally sedated after acupuncture and epilepsy is associated in some individuals with different states of arousal, so it may be possible that the effects of acupuncture could trigger seizures in susceptible animal patients. This is purely supposition: there have been no reports of such a link in the human literature.

(7) Numbers of treatments to determine any change would depend on the baseline seizure pattern.

IMMUNE SYSTEM EFFECTS

There have been great claims made for the effects of acupuncture on the immune system, but the evidence at present is not convincing. A superficial glance at the evidence looks impressive, but it is not conclusive.

Sin in 1983 and Zhou et al. in 1988 demonstrated a positive effect on phagocytic activity[16,17]; an increase in the migration of phagocytic activity was shown by Sliwinsky and Kulej[18], although in the latter experiment the withdrawal of corticosteroids from the patients may help to explain a change in migration. Some studies have shown a positive effect on humoral immunity; others no effect. Cell-mediated immunity has been studied and again some studies have shown, for example, an increase in CD4 and CD11 cells after moxibustion for the treatment of patients with lung cancer[19]. On the other hand a study of needling in rheumatoid arthritis showed no significant changes in the numbers of T lymphocytes, NK cells or immunoglobulin levels[20].

If acupuncture does have a positive effect on the immune system, some studies have given an indication of how that may be mediated. The rate of transformation of lymphocytes was significantly increased over controls in rabbits treated with electroacupuncture, but this effect was not blocked by a neurotoxic agent[21,22]. Since the agent in question blocked the adrenergic mechanisms of the brain, this implies that central catecholamines play some part in the effects of acupuncture on the immune system. This hypothesis was further supported by an experiment in which mice showed a doubling of T-helper lymphocytes after strong manual acupuncture compared with controls, but not if they were first treated with anti-adrenergic drugs[23].

What is important to remember is that the immune system may be affected by many of the non-specific effects of acupuncture. Psychological influences can affect the immune system, as has been demonstrated by cognitive behavioural intervention and hypnotic suggestion[24]. The relatively simple effects of classical (i.e. Pavlovian) conditioning were demonstrated in an experiment on rats, where the rats were given a distinctly flavoured drink along with an immunosuppressant drug. Here the drug is the unconditioned stimulus and the suppression of the immune system the unconditioned response. After the conditioned stimulus of the drink has been administered several times it can alone produce the conditioned response of suppressing the immune system[25]. Therefore it is difficult to demonstrate with confidence specific effects of needling on any aspect of the immune system, since there are many ways by which it might be affected.

A more recent piece of work may illustrate this: in 2003 Karst and his colleagues chose LI11, a point traditionally said to have positive effects on immune function (the canine equivalent is shown in Figure 9.1) to test the effects of real needling compared with sham needling (with the placebo needle) on the respiratory burst of neutrophils. The respiratory burst is part of the neutrophil's mechanism of activating intracellular enzyme systems during which reactive oxygen intermediates are produced. Such intermediates play a major role in the elimination of bacteria and fungi by the neutrophils.

The results showed an increase in respiratory burst in both groups, but more significantly in the group that received the real acupuncture. The authors suggested that psychological effects played a part in the control group who knew that the 'acupuncture' was to affect the immune system. It was also interesting to note that six of the eleven volunteers in the control group experienced *de qi*, or the needling sensation, with the placebo needle. This produces a possible confounding factor in that people feeling *de qi* may also have had a physiological response to the sham needling, although the authors note that three without the needling sensation had marked rises in the measured respiratory burst[26].

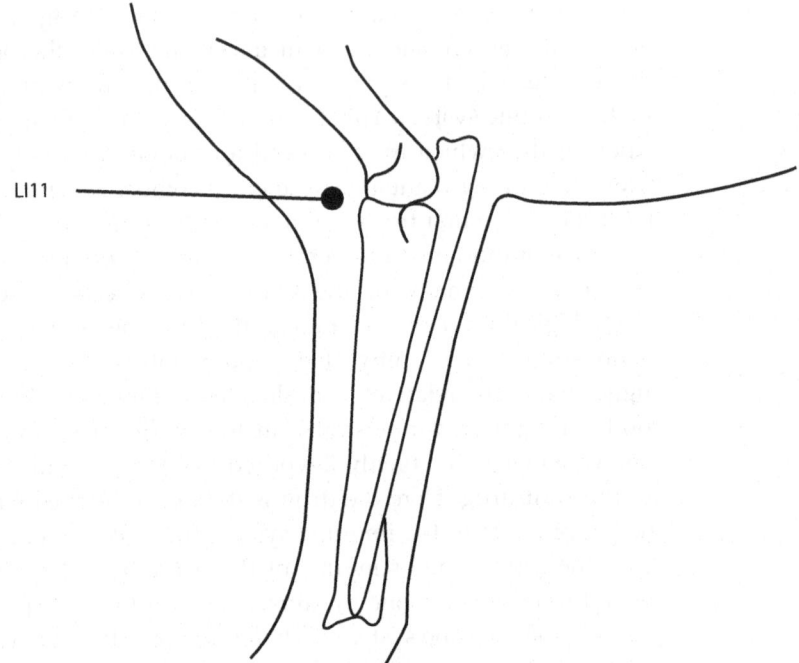

Figure 9.1   LI11 in the dog. LI11 is found halfway between the lateral epicondyle of the humerus and the biceps tendon.

Hypersensitivity reactions

In many ways, positive effects on hypersensitivity reactions would be of greater interest to the general practitioner using acupuncture. Much of the distress, frustration and source of client dissatisfaction is in the treatment of such conditions, especially with corticosteroids, which are seen all too often as a 'bad thing' by pet owners.

There is a limited amount of evidence on delayed-type hypersensitivity in mice. In a study by Kasahara *et al.* electroacupuncture at GV4, a midline point, reduced the swelling produced by a chemical, to which the animals had been sensitised, by 45–73%[27,28]. This result is similar to that obtained by using corticosteroids. This mechanism was shown to depend on the release of opioid peptides and on an intact pituitary gland.

In this experiment it was noted that 'non-specific points' in the femoral muscle had no effect, but it should be remembered that one can be far from confident about transposing acupoints from man to mouse.

This and other studies are fascinating and provide the basis and hypotheses for further studies, but they do not give a lucid and overall view of the effect of acupuncture on the immune system in a clinical setting. Some of the studies have apparently contradictory findings and it cannot be said with confidence that a positive effect on one aspect of the immune system will have predictable and positive effects on the rest when one is dealing with a real clinical case.

Clinical notes

(1) The evidence so far is by no means sufficiently convincing to use acupuncture as a sole method of enhancing immune function where it is compromised, or of damping it down where it is overactive.

(2) Note that care should be taken when needling immunocompromised animals because of an increased risk of infection.

(3) Specific therapies should be used where indicated, but acupuncture could be used as an adjunctive therapy as part of a planned treatment. For example: one may try to attempt to treat an atopic individual showing early Cushingoid changes after protracted use of corticosteroid. Acupuncture should be started well in advance of any slow withdrawal of the corticosteroids. Be aware that some owners may see the use of any therapy such as acupuncture as a legitimate reason to stop the current medication.

(4) There is no evidence to suggest that the overall action of acupuncture is blocked by corticosteroids, although any positive effect on immune function may of course be countered by the steroids themselves, depending on the dose.

(5) Point selection would seem to be non-specific. LI11 is a convenient point in all species and since some positive effects have been demonstrated by treatment at this point it would seem a sensible selection. For a generalised effect, the selection of some midline points (GV points most conveniently in the veterinary species) and bilateral forelimb and hindlimb points that are well tolerated and easy to stimulate either manually or by electroacupuncture would seem the best approach.

(6) Use electroacupuncture or strong manual stimulation if tolerated.

(7) In terms of prognosis, it may be that there is a degree of individual sensitivity, much as there is in response to acupuncture analgesia. It is possible that good responses may be seen in susceptible individuals, but given our current level of evidence it would be unfair and unjust to suggest to owners that the effects

of, say, chemotherapy or radiotherapy, autoimmune disorders or hypersensitivity reactions can be reversed by needling.

NAUSEA AND VOMITING

There is an extensive amount of evidence on the effects of acupuncture in nausea and vomiting in humans. A systematic review by Vickers in 1996 concluded that 11 of 12 of the highest quality trials were positive[29]. This review concluded that stimulation of acupuncture point PC6 in humans seemed to be an effective antiemetic technique, except when administered under general anaesthesia. PC6 was the most common point tested and this is because it has been traditionally used as an antiemetic point. A meta-analysis by Lee and Done concluded that non-pharmacological techniques (including acupuncture, electroacupuncture, transcutaneous electrical nerve stimulation, acupoint stimulation and acupressure) were equivalent to commonly used antiemetics in preventing vomiting after surgery[30]. It also concluded that such techniques were more effective than placebo in preventing nausea and vomiting up to six hours after surgery (but not so-called 'late vomiting') in adults.

Essentially the summary of evidence is that there is an antiemetic effect of acupuncture on postoperative and post-chemotherapy nausea and vomiting and a synergistic effect of acupuncture with antiemetic drugs. The evidence is less convincing overall for the nausea and vomiting associated with pregnancy and travel sickness, although studies tend to suggest that strong stimulation is required for an effect in *hyperemesis gravidum* (severe vomiting associated with pregnancy, usually requiring hospitalisation). It would seem that needling needs to occur around or soon after the emetic stimulus and that may be why the evidence is less convincing in non-hospitalised patients – i.e. those with morning sickness and travel sickness.

Mechanism of antiemesis

Although there is a convincing body of evidence for an effect in humans, there is still no particularly convincing mechanism of action for the antinausea or antiemetic effects of acupuncture. There may be a psychological action, but in a study by Dundee and Ghaly (1991) the antiemetic action was blocked by the injection of the chosen site, PC6, with local anaesthetic[31]. The fact that antiemesis can be achieved by needling before and after anaesthesia, but not during tends to suggest that an intact nervous system is required, as it is for acupuncture analgesia[32-34]. It has been postulated that a different mechanism is involved than that evoked in acupuncture analgesia and the general consensus seems to be against any endorphin-mediated action[35,36].

The vomiting centre, demonstrated by Borison and Wang in 1953, is stimulated from various sites but the chemoreceptor trigger zone, on the floor of the fourth ventricle, senses chemical stimuli[37]. Vomiting occurs when the blood concentration of these chemicals reaches a certain level and the neurotransmitters postulated to be involved include serotonin and dopamine; receptors for cholinergic, adrenergic and antihistaminergic drugs may also be involved[38].

Antiemesis in the veterinary species

How does this relate to the veterinary patient? For dogs, vomiting is often not associated with nausea and their emetic response is much more easily evoked than humans. Horses and ruminants do not vomit (except in very specific and serious conditions, e.g. rhododendron toxicity) and in all veterinary species it is difficult to objectively quantify nausea when it does occur. Excessive salivation in the dog and cat usually indicates nausea, although it is not pathognomonic for nausea (severe anxiety will produce the same effects in dogs, for example, although there is nothing to say that nausea is not involved in that emotion); the consumption of plant material does not always precede vomiting but is often present in dogs who appear to be suffering from dietary sensitivities. Walking away or backing away from food may be a sign of nausea, but may also indicate dental pain or even neck pain. Excessive yawning in horses tends to indicate colic, but colic is just a collection of signs; no one knows whether nausea is involved in colic, but it seems not unreasonable to presume that it may be. Dogs with dietary sensitivities are often seen to yawn excessively (personal observation, SL), although they will yawn too in situations of emotional conflict. Depression generally associated with any toxic condition (e.g. pyometra) may indicate feelings of nausea, but central depression is caused by many factors relating to a diseased state. Many of the studies included in the reviews described above do not distinguish between nausea and vomiting, although some do, therefore we are left with little idea as to whether acupuncture is likely to be useful for one or the other sign in the veterinary patient.

Clinical notes

(1) Where specific treatments are indicated for vomiting these should be used.

(2) Since the evidence is so strong in humans, it seems sensible to try acupuncture as an adjunctive therapy, particularly in refractory cases.

(3) Nausea and vomiting are self-limiting in many disease processes, as long as the disease is dealt with promptly and appropriately, e.g. ovariohysterectomy in pyometra, antibiotic therapy for bacterial gastrointestinal disease. Clearly, acupuncture is not a substitute for such specific therapy, therefore a diagnosis should be reached wherever possible. However, there are some indications for which the practitioner may wish to try any reasonable treatment to reduce nausea and get the patient to eat again. Renal failure is one such case; acupuncture as part of planned palliative care for chronic renal failure in dogs and cats may be a route worth pursuing. So far only anecdotal evidence is available and care should be taken in immunocompromised animals. Treatment would need to be repeated since the emetic stimulus cannot be removed (uraemia), but this may be manageable as part of a therapeutic plan.

(4) Point selection: although PC6 has been tested in most of the studies cited above, it seems unlikely that an antiemetic effect would be point specific. Also, the significance of the lower third of the forearm in humans may be very different both psychologically and physiologically from that of the dog, horse or cat. It is an awkward site in these species, with very little soft tissue to needle and it would seem more logical to choose easily accessible, well tolerated points at which one can stimulate strongly if necessary by manual or electroacupuncture (see Figure 9.2).

(5) More work needs to be done about achieving some kind of objective measurement for nausea in the domestic species. This will probably be more challenging than measuring pain, which is saying something, but the potential suffering associated with nausea is significant. Vomiting is sometimes a protective and useful response – that is of course what it is for – and its absence does not mean that nausea is also absent. Measuring an antiemetic effect is relatively easy, but it would not necessarily indicate success of the treatment for the patient.

BEHAVIOUR PROBLEMS

The fact that acupuncture stimulation causes the release of neurotransmitters such as serotonin and noradrenaline may excite the inter-

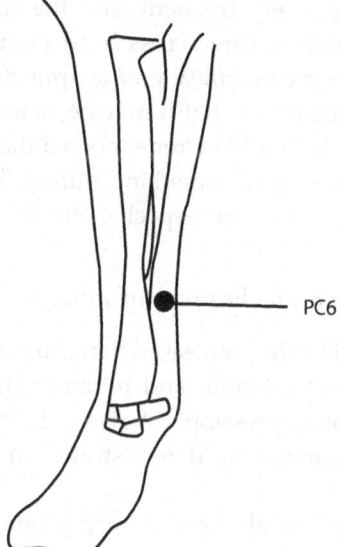

Figure 9.2 PC6 in the dog is located on the caudomedial aspect of the humerus about one third of way between the carpus and the elbow, in the depression between flexor carpi radialis and flexor digitorum profundus.

est of veterinary behaviourists looking for an alternative or an adjunct to psychopharmacy. Behaviour-modifying drugs for our companion animals tend to be serotonergic, dopaminergic or, off-licence, noradrenergic, in their main actions and all have the potential for serious side effects, either behaviourally, physically or both. In the problem of compulsive behaviours one may be looking for all or some of these effects as well as an endorphin-mediated response, depending on the time frame of the condition. The situation is not clear-cut. Add that to the paucity of information on the use of acupuncture for psychological problems in humans (where the psychological effects of receiving any treatment could be significantly different from that of animals) and the conclusion is that acupuncture should not be considered as a substitute for treatment for behavioural disorders.

Treatment of depression in humans

Three studies from the Institute of Mental Health in Beijing demonstrated that acupuncture was as useful as amitriptyline (a common tricyclic anti-depressant) in the treatment of depression of mixed aetiology and depressive psychosis[39–41]. Treatment frequency ranged from 30 one-hour sessions over five weeks to daily treatments for six weeks, i.e. very frequent, and the stimulation in all cases involved electroacupuncture across head points. The studies do not demonstrate a specific efficacy of acupuncture in the treatment of depression, but suggest that it may be as useful as the usual antidepressant therapy. It should be remembered that patients would also be having an interaction of some kind during the intense therapy sessions and this may have a non-specific effect.

Supposed mechanism of action

In 1986 Han hypothesised that acupuncture accelerated synthesis and release of serotonin and noradrenaline and that this could explain effects on depression[42]. A rise in L5 hydroxytryptophan (a precursor of serotonin) was demonstrated in rabbits in 1974 by Chein and Zakaira[43].

While this all sounds very promising, it should be remembered that, although antidepressants cause a rise in serotonin and noradrenaline, among other neurotransmitters, it is the secondary messenger effects induced by these transmitters that produce the clinical effect. The neurotransmitter levels need to be maintained at a sufficient level over two to three weeks to induce these effects, which is why there is a delay in action of such drugs when there is no delay in the effect on neurotransmitters. In other words, just increasing mood neurotransmitters for a few hours or few days (or few minutes) after acupuncture is not likely to be sufficient to give a clinical effect. It may be reasonable to expect some real effect from strong, daily electroacupuncture over five or six weeks, as in the studies described, but perhaps not from brief weekly needling, except in very sensitive individuals.

Clinical notes

(1) Behaviour therapy is effective in many cases of behavioural disorders and antidepressant therapy is not a necessary first line treatment in most cases[44].

(2) Clinical causes of behaviour problems should be ruled out wherever possible. In the experience of one of the authors (SL clinical audit) pain may account for up to 25% of behaviour problems. Acupuncture may be a useful treatment for these cases, but identification of such pain would be useful if one is not to erroneously credit acupuncture with miraculous results for behaviour problems.

(3) If an animal is considered to be sufficiently disturbed to require behaviour modifying drugs then specific treatments in the form of medication or pheromone therapy should be used. Acupuncture could be used adjunctively as part of a planned therapeutic regime, either where the side effects of the medication are considered a contraindication to its use or where sufficient effect is not achieved.

(4) The evidence and our knowledge about the action of antidepressants suggest that acupuncture treatment may need to be so frequent as to be impractical in a clinical setting and few animals are going to tolerate prolonged electroacupuncture treatment across the head.

(5) Practically then, as an adjunct or treatment in refractory cases, acupuncture should be given twice weekly if possible for the first three weeks. Strong manual stimulation or, preferably, electroacupuncture should be used at a frequency of 80–100 Hz (or dense dispersed at 2 Hz and 80–100 Hz – see Chapter 11).

(6) Point selection: it is probably not necessary to use head points and it is difficult to keep the needles in place during electroacupuncture in this position. Neurotransmitter release due to acupuncture is not limited to the use of points on the head, so general, easily accessible and well-tolerated points can be chosen.

(7) Beware of owners withdrawing tricyclic antidepressant medication suddenly.

SUMMARY

Acupuncture may have a positive effect on non-painful conditions, but the possible mechanisms of action are unclear. In some cases, such as nausea and vomiting in humans, the level of evidence for an effect in a clinical setting is as convincing, or more so, than that for analgesia in chronic pain. All the work on animals is experimental and, while that may provide us with useful starting points for hypothesising action and likely effect, it does not provide the clinician with any firm guidance as to likely effectiveness. For most of the conditions described, acupuncture may be used as an adjunctive therapy, general or favourite points chosen and robust stimulation applied. The identification of outcome measures is essential if one is going to use acupuncture as part of a planned therapeutic regime.

REFERENCES

1. Rees JR, Laidlaw A. Pruritus: more scratch than itch. *Clin Exp Dermatol* 1999;24:490–3.
2. Schmelz M, Schmidt R, Bickel A. Specific C receptors for itch in human skin. *J Neurosci* 1997;17:8003–8.
3. Belgrade MJ, Solomon LM, Lichter EA. Effect of acupuncture on experimentally induced itch. *Acta Derm Venereol (Stockh)* 1984;64:129–33.
4. Lundeberg T, Bondesson L, Thomas M. Effect of acupuncture on experimentally induced itch. *Br J Dermatol* 1987;117:771–7.
5. Duo LJ. Electrical needle therapy of uraemic pruritus. *Nephron* 1987;47(3):179–83.
6. Lundeberg T, Kjartansson J, Samuelson U. Effect of electrical nerve stimulation on healing of ischaemic skin flaps. *Lancet* 1988;2(8613):712–14.
7. Jansen G, Lundeberg T, Samuelson UE, Thomas M. Increased survival of ischaemic musculocutaneous flaps in rats after acupuncture. *Acta Physiol Scand* 1989;135:555–8.
8. Jansen G, Lundeberg T, Kjartsson J, Samuelson UE. Acupuncture and sensory neuropeptides increase cutaneous blood flow in rats. *Neurosci Lett* 1989;97:305–9.
9. Dawidson I, Blom M, Lundeberg T, Angmar-Mansson B. The influence of acupuncture treatment on the release of neuropeptides in saliva in healthy subjects. *Caries Res* 1993;S32.
10. Sterner-Victorin E, Lundeberg T, Waldenstrom U, Manni L, Aloe L, Gunnarsson S. Effects of electro-acupuncture on nerve growth factor and ovarian morphology in rats with experimentally induced polycystic ovaries. *Biol Reprod* 2000;63(5):1497–503.
11. Walton DK. Psychodermatoses. In: Kirk RW, editor. *Current Veterinary Therapy IX: Small Animal Practice*. Philadelphia: WB Saunders; 1986. pp. 557–92.
12. Veith L. Acral lick dermatitis in the dog. *Canine Pract* 1986;13:15–22.
13. Paterson S. A placebo-controlled study to investigate clomipramine in the treatment of canine lick granuloma. In: Kwocha KW, Willemse T, and von Tscharner C, editors. *Advances in Veterinary Dermatology, 5th edn.* Philadelphia: WB Saunders; 1995. pp. 845–58.
14. Janssens LAA. Ear acupuncture for treatment of epilepsy in the dog. *Progr Vet Neurol* 1993;4(3):89–94.
15. Panzer RB, Chrisman CL. An auricular acupuncture for idiopathic canine epilepsy: a preliminary report. *Am J Chin Med* 1994;22(1):11–17.
16. Sin YM. Effect of electric acupuncture and moxibustion on phagocytic activity of the reticulo-endothelial system of mice. *Am J Acupunct* 1983;11(3):237–41.
17. Zhou R, Huang F, Jiang S, Jiang J. The effect of acupuncture on the phagocytic activity of human leucocytes. *J Tradit Chin Med* 1988;8(2):83–4.

18. Sliwinski J, Kulej M. Acupuncture induced immunoregulatory influence on the clinical state of patients suffering from chronic spastic bronchitis and undergoing long-term treatment with corticosteroids. *Acupunct Electrother Res* 1989;14:227–34.

19. Ouyang Q, Cao M, Cao Q. An observation on the effect of moxibustion on the immunological functions in 69 cases of lung cancer. *Int J Clin Acupunct* 1992;3(4):369–73.

20. Liu X, Sun L, Xiao JI. Effects of acupuncture and point function in rheumatoid arthritis. *J Tradit Chin Med* 1993;13(3):174–8.

21. Zhao J, Liu W. Relationship between acupuncture induced immunity and the regulation of central neurotransmitter system in rabbits: I Effect of central catecholaminergic neurons in regulating acupuncture-induced immune function. *Acupunct Electrother Res* 1988;13:79–85.

22. Zhao J, Liu W. Relationship between acupuncture induced immunity and the regulation of central neurotransmitter system in rabbits: II Effect of the endogenous opioid peptides on the regulation of acupuncture-induced immune reaction. *Acupunct Electrother Res* 1989;14:1–7.

23. Lundeberg T, Eriksson SV, Theodorsson E. Neuroimmunomodulatory effects of acupuncture in mice. *Neurosci Lett* 1991;128:161–4.

24. Kiecolt-Glaser JK, Glaser R. Psychoneuroimmunology: can psychological interventions modulate immunity? *J Consult Clin Psychol* 1992;60:569–75.

25. Ader R, Cohen N, Felten D. Psychoneuroimmunology: interactions between the nervous system and the immune system. *Lancet* 1995; 345:99–103.

26. Karst M, Scheinichen D, Rueckert T, Wagner T, Wiese B, Piepenbrock S, Fink M. Effect of acupuncture on the neutrophil respiratory burst: a placebo-controlled single blinded study. *Complement Ther Med* 2003;11: 4–10.

27. Kasahara T, Wu Y, Sakurai Y, Oguchi K. Suppressive effect of acupuncture on delayed type hypersensitivity to trinitrochlorobenzene and involvement of opiate receptors. *Int J Immunopharmacol* 1992;14(4): 661–5.

28. Kasahara T, Amemiya M, Wu Y, Oguchi K. Involvement of central opioidergic and nonopioidegic neuroendocrine systems in the suppressive effect of acupuncture on delayed type hypersensitivity in mice. *Int J Immunopharmacol* 1993;15(4):501–8.

29. Vickers AJ. Can acupuncture have specific effects on health? A systematic review of acupuncture anti emesis trials. *J R Soc Med* 1996;89(6):303–11.

30. Lee A, Done ML. The use of non-pharmacologic techniques to prevent post operative nausea and vomiting: a meta analysis. *Anaesth Analg* 1999;88(6):1362–9.

31. Dundee JW, Ghaly RG. Local anaesthesia blocks the antiemetic action of P6 acupuncture. *Clin Pharmacol Ther* 1991;50:78–80.

32. Dundee JW, Ghaly RG, Bill KM, Chestnutt WM, Fitzpatrick KTJ, Lynas AGA. Effect of stimulation of the P6 antiemetic point on postoperative nausea and vomiting. *Br J Anaesth* 1989;63:612–18.

33. Ho RT, Jawan B, Fung ST, Cheung HK, Lee JH. Electroacupuncture and postoperative emesis. *Anaesthesia* 1990;45(4):327–9.

34. Weightman WM, Zacharias M, Herbison P. Traditional Chinese acupuncture as an emetic. *BMJ* 1987;295:1379–80.

35. Lenhard L, White PME. Acupuncture in the prophylactic treatment of migraine headaches: pilot study. *N Z Med J* 1983;96:663–6.

36. Harris AL. Cytotoxic-therapy induced vomiting is mediated via enkephalic pathways. *Lancet* 1982;i:714–16.

37. Borison HL, Wang SG. Physiology and pharmacology of vomiting. *Pharmacol Rev* 1953;5:193–230.

38. Borison HL, McCarthy LE. Neuropharmacology of chemotherapy-induced emesis. *Drugs* 1983;25(Suppl 1):8–17.

39. Luo HC, Jia YK, Li Z. Electroacupuncture vs amitryptiline in the treatment of depressive states. *J Tradit Chin Med* 1985;5:3–8.

40. Yang X. Clinical observation on needling extrachannel points in treating mental depression. *J Tradit Chin Med* 1994;14:14–18.

41. Lou H, Jia Y, Wu X, Dai W. Electroacupuncture in the treatment of depressive psychosis. A controlled prospective randomized trial using electro-acupuncture and amitryptiline in 241 patients. *Int J Clin Acupunct* 1990;1:7–13.

42. Han JS. Electroacupuncture: an alternative to antidepressants for treating affective diseases? *Int J Neurosci* 1986;29:79–92.

43. Chein EYM, Zakaira S. Acupuncture for psychiatric disorders. *JAMA* 1974;229:639.

44. Scott S, Mayhew IG. Guest Editorial: pharmacological treatment in behavioural medicine. *Vet J* 2001;162(1):5–6.

Part Three

Practical aspects of acupuncture in the veterinary species

NEEDLES

Modern acupuncture needles are usually made from stainless steel, although some practitioners with a traditional bent may still use gold or silver needles for their purported special properties. From the Western perspective stainless steel fulfils the following criteria:

(1) It is relatively cheap: 1000 needles cost anything from £2.50 to £14.00 depending on brand and supplier, but, at a maximum of 14 pence per needle, it is neither difficult nor prohibitive to include the equipment costs in the price of a treatment.

(2) It can be manufactured to a high standard in terms of smoothness at the tip. Although even the best needles can be demonstrated under electronmicroscopy to have occasional imperfections that could snag on soft tissue, needles can be made to be smooth enough to penetrate without the patient noticing. Some medical practitioners like the slightly spiky nature of some needles, because they feel that it adds to the *de qi* and provides a bigger afferent stimulation, but this also means that they are more uncomfortable when inserted. While this may be acceptable to some, if not all, human patients, our veterinary patients are unlikely to be as sanguine in their response. After all, most are already expecting an uncomfortable procedure because of their previous experiences in a clinic.

(3) Stainless steel needles can be manufactured to a degree that means that, despite bending and twisting, they are highly unlikely to

153

break. Many dogs will suddenly lie down during a treatment and may lean on their needles. Mostly these needles just come out, but sometimes they bend. More dramatically, needles inserted into the epaxial muscles of the horse, and sometimes the dog, will come out twisted into a corkscrew shape or bent at nearly right angles because of the contraction of the muscles into which they were inserted. The first time this is experienced is usually the last time one considers using needles of lower quality.

(4) Stainless steel needles can be sterilised. Modern practice recommends the use of single use, disposable, sterile needles, disposed of after use into the standard sharps bins.

Presentation of needles

Needles are packed in a variety of ways:

(1) *Packed singly with a guide tube* and one of several methods of holding the needle within the tube until ready for insertion. The guide tube is a hollow, rigid, plastic cylinder within which fits the needle. The needle can be held in place with a piece of plastic, which can be removed before insertion, or a spot weld of plastic attaching the needle handle to the guide tube. This weld needs to be broken before use. These methods of fixing the needle prevent it falling out of the guide tube as it is removed from the sterile packet. The needle is fixed in the guide tube such that the sharp end is within the tube, as illustrated in Figure 10.1. These features enhance safety, but the guide tube is primarily used to guide the needle during insertion. The needles are very fine and can bend during insertion; the guide tube provides a rigid framework until the first few millimetres of the needle have penetrated the dermis. The tube also provides some pressure on the skin to distract the patient from the sharp prick of insertion. For human patients, the use of a guide tube also prevents them seeing the initial insertion of the needle; this is useful in nervous patients. However, it is worth noting the following about using guide tubes in the veterinary species: the first insertion of the needle through the tube allows the needle to penetrate only a few millimetres, just below the dermis. The tube is then removed and the needle pushed in further to the required depth. If the patient is fractious or agitated then the first insertion may cause sharp movement resulting in the needle being flicked out of the skin once the tube is removed. In other words, the veterinarian should be confident of having

two chances to insert the needle, otherwise it is preferable to use no guide tube. In horses particularly, the insertion of a needle sub-dermally may provoke a strong reaction that resembles the patient being bitten by flies: the skin may twitch violently, the horse may turn to grab at the needles and may become fractious and difficult to restrain. This reaction is not consistent in horses, but is worth being aware of and this author (SL) would use no guide tube when treating horses except when inserting long needles or if the horse is well restrained or sedated.

(2) *Packed in multiples with one guide tube.* This is a more economical way of packaging, but does mean that the needle must be inserted into the guide tube before it can be used and is therefore time-consuming. Sheathing or re-sheathing needles carries the risk of needle-stick injuries.

(3) *Packed singly or in multiples with no guide tube.* Many practitioners do not use guide tubes. The usual technique of insertion in this case is to tense the skin on either side of the insertion site and to insert the needle quickly. It is worth getting used to the technique of needle insertion without guide tubes so that horses can be treated more easily (see 1 above) and so that the same needle can be used, if desired, on the same patient (in the same session) for multiple insertions without the time-consuming and potentially risky procedure of re-sheathing the needle.

Size of needle

These generally range from 0.16 mm in diameter to 0.4 mm in diameter, and from 0.5 mm in length to 75 mm in length. The difference in sensation between the finest and thickest is considerable; choice of length depends upon the species treated and the depth required to reach the desired point or tissue.

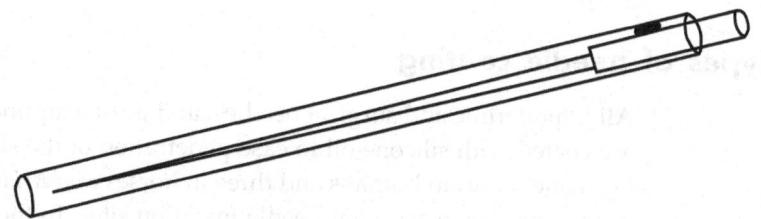

Figure 10.1 Needle in the guide tube. The needle is kept within the guide tube until the spot weld is broken.

The reader should by now have realised that there are no hard and fast rules in acupuncture, but a general guide is:

- 0.16 mm × 30 mm needles are used for cats, rabbits and sensitive or hyperalgesic dogs.
- Alternatively, because long needles may easily fall out in animals with little subcutaneous tissue, 0.2 mm × 20 mm or even shorter could be used in cats and rabbits.
- 0.25 mm × 40 mm needles are used for dogs and many sites in horses.
- 0.3 mm × 50 mm or 75 mm needles are used for deeper sites in horses and larger mammals. These long needles are difficult to insert and usually require a series of cut down guide tubes to stop the needle bending excessively.

Depending on the animals most commonly treated it is possible to keep a reasonable stock of just two or three sizes of needles, rather than feeling that every size and length should be kept 'just in case' and then finding that they have outlived their shelf life.

Type of handle

Handles are either plastic or metal. There is no particular reason to choose one over the other except when considering the use of electroacupuncture. Metal handled needles are required for electroacupuncture so that the electrodes can be attached to an electroconducting material. It is feasible to use the shaft of the needle for this, depending on the clips in use, but it can be fiddly and it should be remembered that the clips are not sterilised after use (see: Chapter 11).

From an 'alternative' point of view, it has been mentioned that metal handles are superior because they allow transfer of so-called 'energy' between therapist and patient, but from the neurophysiological perspective there is no evidence to suggest that this is the case.

Types of needle coating

All hypodermic and surgical needles, and most acupuncture needles, are coated with silicone oil to ease penetration of the skin. There has been one report in humans and three in horses *worldwide*, of a silicone granulomatous reaction at needle insertion sites. In these cases, particles of silicone were deposited subcutaneously and a foreign body type reaction resulted[1,2].

Such reports have been used to suggest that silicon-coated acupuncture needles should not be used and alternatives have been produced; for those concerned there are needles available with paraben coating. Be aware, however, that if your patient is susceptible to silicon oil, then it is likely to react after the use of standard hypodermic needles or surgical instruments as well as after acupuncture.

Stimulation of the needles

In traditional terms, the way in which needles are moved in the body once they have been inserted is important and depends upon the diagnosis made. Terms such as 'sedate' and 'tonify' are used in traditional terminology and how one achieves these depends on the direction of rotation, insertion or stimulation (depending on which text is consulted) of the needle. From a neurophysiological perspective: more vigorous stimulation of the needles achieves more afferent input. However, more is not always better and the clinician should be careful not to cause C fibre pain (soreness) instead of A delta fibre stimulation since the aim is to produce A delta stimulation to compete with the existing C fibre pain, not to make the patient feel more unpleasant pain. A more robust stimulus is usually achieved by a technique called lift and thrust, which is better demonstrated than described, and involves lifting the needle slightly and advancing it again, sometimes subtly redirecting the needle tip. It is worth noting that rotation of the needle (i.e. spinning it between the finger and thumb as shown in Figures 10.2 and 10.3) may have very little added effect if the needles are very smooth.

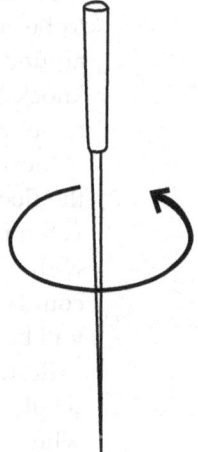

Figure 10.2 Rotation of the needle in the direction of the flow of Qi is traditionally said to achieve tonification of the point.

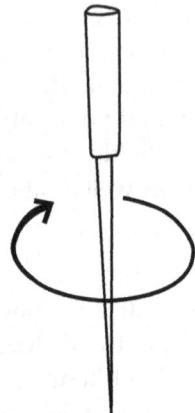

Figure 10.3 Rotation of the needle against the direction of flow of Qi is traditionally said to achieve sedation of the point.

Some veterinary acupuncture practitioners do not stimulate the needles at all because animals tend to shift about during treatment much more than human patients and thereby stimulate the needles themselves.

Stronger stimulation of the needle can be achieved by applying an electrical current between two needles from an electrical impulse generator. This technique is known as electroacupuncture and will be described in greater detail in Chapter 11.

RESTRAINT

Restraint: small animals

Most animals accept acupuncture remarkably well. Some barely need to be restrained at all, although, if patients are allowed to wander around the consulting room, this will result in lost needles as they knock against the walls and as muscle movements cause the needles to be worked outwards.

Most dogs from collie size upwards are probably better treated on the floor, although this will depend to a large extent on whether the veterinarian is fit enough to spend time on the floor and still arise with a modicum of dignity and without sounding as though they could do with much the same treatment. Small dogs, cats and rabbits will be more easily treated on the table.

Restraint should be gentle, but firm to start with; a good guide would be to use the same restraint as required for that individual when administering a subcutaneous injection, although it is likely that the acceptance of the acupuncture needles will be better. If the dog requires muzzling for normal procedures, then start the acupuncture treatment with it muzzled.

Although it is easier for most conditions to start with the patient standing, it is not unusual for them to sit or lie down during treatment. Struggling with them to keep them upright will probably result in more needles being lost than if they are allowed to gently sit or lie. The main caveats here are that one should know where the needle tips are and where they will go if driven in; needles should not be left in place in the ventral surface in case animals do suddenly lie down and, although lying down on the side is usually fine, rolling onto the back if there are needles in the back muscles is best avoided.

Restraint: large animals

Again, the commonsense approach is best: use the usual restraint for a similar procedure such as injection.

Sedation and general anaesthesia

There is no reason to avoid sedation when performing acupuncture except that it will increase the cost to the client and increase the time total treatment takes. It may also mean that an individual needs to be sedated once a week; a notion that many owners will not like. In general one should take a balanced view: if the animal is suffering from a condition that is likely to respond to acupuncture but needs sedation, then do so as long as it is clinically safe for that individual.

The main cited reason for avoiding sedation is that it will interfere with the effect of the acupuncture. The evidence for this is equivocal, but there are some indications from the literature. In 1991 Eriksson *et al.* showed that the effect of low frequency electroacupuncture was reduced if diazepam was used as a sedative agent[3]. In 1983 Xu *et al.* had shown that both diazepam and ketamine antagonised the effects of acupuncture analgesia in rabbits[4]. Having said that, the same study indicated that a number of compounds potentiated the analgesic effects of acupuncture: these included fentanyl and pethidine. Kho *et al.* in 1991 used diazepam and low dose opioids as premedicating agents for acupuncture analgesia and found the results to be satisfactory[5]. In practice then avoiding partial opiate antagonists and ketamine may be sensible until more work is available. Acupuncture appears to work through many different mechanisms and is not likely to be completely blocked by a single chemical factor.

However, deep general anaesthesia is likely to interfere with the centrally mediated mechanisms of acupuncture. It is sensible to treat as the animal starts to come round from the anaesthesia or before induction if treating for perioperative pain or if wanting to treat for a condition that the clinician has just identified under anaesthesia and radiography, e.g. osteoarthritis. The possible exception to this is the treatment of trigger points. Since we still do not know for certain why acupuncture seems to be so effective for the deactivation of trigger points it is impossible to say with confidence that general anaesthesia will not interfere with their treatment, but if at least part of the mechanism involves a direct influence on the affected muscle then it is likely that needling under anaesthesia will deactivate the trigger point. There are advantages to this: if, for example, radiography reveals no bony changes or abnormalities, but there are significantly large or active (there may still be a pain response under anaesthesia to pressure on the trigger point) trigger points then treatment can be started at once. The needling of trigger points can be very uncomfortable, if not actually painful and many animals will resist and resent direct needling of the points. General anaesthesia allows the clinician to locate accurately the taut band and to insert the needle directly.

To summarise the use of chemical restraint in acupuncture

(1) General anaesthesia should not be used simply to facilitate acupuncture treatment.
(2) If acupuncture is to be given during general anaesthesia then it should be done as the anaesthesia starts to wear off or pre-induction depending on what one is trying to achieve.
(3) Identification and treatment of trigger points during general anaesthesia does appear to be a valid and useful approach.
(4) Sedation can be used to help restrain fractious or very anxious patients. Remember that in these cases the animal will not learn to accept the acupuncture because sedation causes a block of the so-called 'short-term memory'.
(5) Sedation can be used if the animal is showing signs of hyperalgesia or allodynia and is consequently in too much pain to needle.
(6) If the acupuncture treatment works then the central sensitisation should decrease and, as the hyperalgesia becomes less pronounced, it should be possible to progress to acupuncture without sedation.

(7) The clinician's preferred sedation can be used, but for maximum effect of the acupuncture, anything that includes a partial opiate antagonist or ketamine may be best avoided, although there is no direct evidence that these interfere with acupuncture in practice.

The use of the twitch in horses

The use of the twitch to pacify or merely restrain horses for procedures is a controversial one. It has been shown to result in elevated levels of endorphins and has been compared to acupuncture for that reason[6]. This is a little simplistic since many stimuli cause release of endorphins including, of course, very painful ones. The twitch may also work via diffuse noxious inhibitory control (DNIC) in which a profoundly painful stimulus at one site in the body can produce widespread analgesia in other areas of the body[7]. The twitch response does appear to be an individual one however and many horses do appear very relaxed while twitched. However, others resist twitching strongly and some are more fractious when twitched than not. The question here is whether or not twitching a horse could interfere with acupuncture treatment. On the one hand the fact that endorphins are released could mean that acupuncture may be enhanced or facilitated by the use of the twitch, on the other, if the animal is focused on a profound afferent stimulus being applied to its muzzle it may have little attention to give to a tiny needle prick elsewhere.

Evidence from Chung et al. in 1984 showed that increasing the level of stimulation to recruit C fibres and thereby raising the intensity of stimulation above the pain threshold does produce some additional analgesia, but this is likely to involve other mechanisms such as DNIC and the welfare implications of causing more pain in the hope of a small overall improvement in analgesia would mean that this is unlikely to be a popular, or tolerated, technique in the absence of some good evidence that it has practical, clinical value[8].

It may be sensible, therefore, to avoid twitching in combination with acupuncture until we have more evidence, or to only use it on those animals who display a profoundly relaxed response.

CONCURRENT THERAPY

There is no need to withdraw concurrent therapy when acupuncture treatment is started. There is no evidence that any medication will have an adverse effect on the treatment, although it has often been mentioned that corticosteroids and even non-steroidal anti-inflammatory drugs interfere with the action. From a neurophysiological perspective, there is no reason to believe that this is the case.

Ethical considerations

In any case, withdrawing pain relief before treatment is arguably unethical if one feels that the animal requires analgesia. It may be that the acupuncture will not work in that individual or will not provide sufficient analgesia or will not start working effectively for two to three weeks.

ASSESSMENT OF TREATMENT

Of course, the maintenance of concurrent therapy will make it difficult to assess the effect of the acupuncture treatment. Sometimes we just have to live with that; other times it is necessary to assess which treatment appears to be working better. For example, a dog with osteoarthritis may be on a programme of non-steroidal anti-inflammatory drugs, a glucosamine and chondroitin supplement, weekly hydrotherapy and acupuncture. Each treatment may have been started within weeks of the other, but each may have a delay of onset of clinical improvement. If the patient appears relatively pain free and active then it will be impossible to say which treatment is working, whether they are all working independently or synergistically and whether stopping one would have an adverse effect on the animal's wellbeing. If there are no complicating factors to suggest that non-steroidal anti-inflammatory drugs are contraindicated, then it can be justified to maintain all therapies, altering each as a plateau of improvement is reached. For example: the hydrotherapy treatment may be stopped or reduced in frequency after a six week course; if the patient continues to do well it does not mean that the hydrotherapy played no part in achieving its pain-free state. Equally, one expects acupuncture to have a cumulative effect, so reducing the frequency of treatment to once a month and still maintaining analgesia does not indicate a lack of effect. It may be frustrating not to know which is most effective, but it is not uncommon and perhaps, from a pragmatic viewpoint, it does not much matter so long as none of treatments carries unacceptable risks.

On the other hand, if one is attempting to treat an atopic and pruritic dog with acupuncture in order to reduce or withdraw the need for corticosteroids then quite clearly the steroids will need to be withdrawn at some stage in order to test the effect of the needling. In this case the pattern of treatment would be:

(1) If corticosteroids abolish the pruritus completely, then establish from the history and the records the average time before the itch starts to return (if a depot injection of corticosteroids is used) or the dose and frequency of tablets that just allows the itch to return. Start on the normal pruritus abolishing dose and begin acupuncture four to six weeks before the effect of corticosteroids would be expected to wear off or the itch return as the dose is safely reduced. This should give a realistic amount of time for a clinical effect of the acupuncture to be demonstrated if it is going to work.
(2) If corticosteroids do not completely abolish the itch, then start acupuncture at the normal dose of steroids to achieve the best effect and monitor over weekly treatments for four to six weeks. If there appears to be an improvement then the dose of steroids can be reduced once the best effect of the acupuncture (i.e. a plateau) has been achieved.
(3) In both cases treatment should be continued weekly until the patient has been off the corticosteroids completely for a month, before reducing the frequency of treatments.

So the general rule is to start acupuncture treatment and maintain the concurrent therapy. Once an improvement over and above that attributed to the concurrent therapy is observed, or if four to six weeks of acupuncture has been given, a trial of reduction of the concurrent therapy can begin, *if* in the clinician's opinion it is appropriate to do so. It should not be the clinician's goal to withdraw all other therapy, but to achieve the best result for the patient with the minimum of complications. Beware of the fact that a few owners may have a firm agenda to take their pet off all medication and use acupuncture as a true 'alternative'.

CLINICAL ASPECTS

The individual response

There is no given dose rate for acupuncture in the way that there is a dose rate for medication. For example:

Three 'lift and thrusts' of a 0.3 mm × 30 mm needle in the longissimus muscle of a 40-kg Labrador over ten minutes cannot, as it stands, be said to be either a sufficient or a large or a small dose. In one individual this may be a massive dose, may cause stimulation of C fibres and result in the animal being sore for a day or so after treatment. In another patient this may be no more stimulating than blowing softly at them.

The response to acupuncture appears to be highly individual and largely unpredictable. To some extent a judgement is made at the time of treatment by the *reaction* of the animal. If the animal becomes immediately and profoundly sedated upon insertion of the needles, it will probably be very sensitive to treatment, will need little needle stimulation and will have a good clinical response. An animal that barely seems to notice the needles being inserted may need, and will probably tolerate, stronger stimulation.

The exception to this is the direct needling of trigger points. Most animals will find direct needling of trigger points painful and may even try to snap or bite. This does not necessarily reflect their response to the rest of the acupuncture needling. For this reason one of the authors (SL) does not aim to directly needle trigger points on the first treatment, but allows the animal to accept, and sometimes even apparently enjoy, the treatment.

Responsiveness of the population

There seem to be between 10 and 20% of dogs (SL audit) and people who do not appear to respond to acupuncture at all[9].

There seem to be between 10 and 20% of dogs that appear to be very sensitive to acupuncture and respond dramatically well to minimal treatment (e.g. brief needling).

The middle of 60–80% of patients appear to range from being very sensitive to not very sensitive and need their treatments adjusted accordingly.

Dogs appear to respond to acupuncture in similar ways to human patients, but other species appear to be more sensitive. This is only an anecdotal observation, but it would seem logical to suppose that a prey species, such as the horse, or a highly reactive species such as the cat, would respond more profoundly to an afferent stimulus, particularly one that mimicked real or potential tissue damage.

General rules

(1) Avoid direct and vigorous needling of trigger points on first treatment (although sometimes it is difficult to avoid hitting them and it is worth warning the owner that the animal may react adversely if this happens).

(2) Start with points that seem always to be well tolerated until an impression of the animal's reaction is gauged.

(3) Profound reactions such as dramatic sedation usually indicate sensitivity to treatment and minimal stimulation and short duration of treatment is indicated.

(4) Otherwise assume that an individual is in the middle of the range of sensitivity and treat with some stimulation (three to five movements of each needle) over ten to fifteen minutes.

(5) Soreness and stiffness after treatment indicate that the needling was too robust for that individual so for the next treatment stimulate the needles less and leave in for a shorter time. Continuing soreness post-treatment may indicate the need for the use of finer needles and brief treatment.

(6) No response to treatment would indicate the need for stronger stimulation, needling of trigger points (in musculoskeletal and other painful conditions) and possible use of electroacupuncture.

Frequency of treatment

Unless an animal is very sensitive to treatment, weekly acupuncture is convenient and appears to be sufficiently frequent to produce a cumulative response to treatment. It has been suggested that biweekly treatment, at least for the first two weeks, is optimal, but usual appointment scheduling makes once a week more viable for most practitioners. Daily treatment is usually unnecessary and may be counter-productive.

A course of acupuncture usually consists of four to six treatments one week apart. The owner should be aware of the commitment before they start, but should also be aware that the animal is not necessarily going to be 'better' at the end of this course. This is just a preliminary course to see if and how well the patient responds to acupuncture. Thereafter, the treatment can be spaced out according to maintenance of response.

Treatment times

Twenty minutes of acupuncture is given as the ideal treatment time, although there seems to be no good reason for this beyond tradition. In practice, anything from a brief technique, whereby each needle is inserted, stimulated and then immediately withdrawn, to a fifteen-minute session is acceptable and appears to give results. Many animals seem to start getting restless after ten minutes and, if the needles have become subcutaneous, they will often shake, spraying needles down shirtfronts and under cupboards, which, while it has the merit of entertainment for the owner, does represent a potential sharps hazard and is time-consuming in searching and accounting for all needles. (For this reason, even if needles are easy to see when they are in the patient, needle packets and tubes should be retained to count and compare with the numbers of needles retrieved from the floor and hair.)

There is little merit in forgetting a patient either. In any case, during needling owners should not be left alone with their animals, except for brief periods (see Safety, page 13). During electroacupuncture, treatment times extending beyond 45 minutes result in the release of cholecystokinin octapeptide (CCK-8) from the brain, which, as an opioid antagonist starts to reverse the effects of acupuncture[10]. Once again, more is not always better when it comes to acupuncture.

Reactions to treatment

Note the distinction here between reaction and response. Reaction covers the way in which the animal behaves during or after the treatment; response refers to clinical improvement in symptoms.

During treatment

Reactions vary between individuals. Some animals behave no differently than they would during any other consultation. Others may sit or lie down and look relaxed. Some get a distinctly far way or 'spaced-out' look and often a drip of moisture appears at the end of the nose; some salivate more than usual. Some sensitive individuals will fall asleep or sink to the ground as though sedated. Occasionally, patients will seem more restless than usual and shift or prance about and make it generally difficult to keep the needles in. This may simply be the reaction of an individual to being in the vet's surgery for longer than usual without anything much being done or it may be that some animals start to feel sedated but fight it; the veterinary clinic is after all not likely to be perceived as a safe place to fall asleep. Whether this could ever be interpreted as a genuine euphoria, as is sometimes reported, is another matter. Fortunately, for it is a nuisance, it does not happen very often.

If a trigger point is directly needled or a needle is inserted clumsily or in a very tender area, the animal will react in the same way as it might to any other sudden pain. However, even nice dogs may try to snap or bite when trigger points are targeted, so approach these areas with caution. The animal should not be reprimanded for such a response, but needling should be done at another site or not at all until it has calmed down. Animals may jump when a tender point is first needled but then quickly settle, however if they continue to be agitated and to turn towards the needle then it should be removed. Causing C fibre pain (unpleasant pain, the pain of suffering) is not the intention during acupuncture, although it sometimes is unavoidable.

Areas of hyperalgesia or allodynia can be needled if the animal will tolerate it, but finer needles may need to be used than for other sites. Otherwise it is possible to needle on either side of the sensitive area (a perisegmental approach). The changes that occur in the central nervous system as a response to acupuncture, resulting in the reduction of central sensitisation, will be triggered by needling away from the site of pain as well as locally. When the allodynia is resolved then local needling can occur.

After treatment

Many animals will either sleep in the car or when they get home. Owners report this sleep to be deep, relaxed and longer lasting than they would expect. Some animals still appear sleepy the next day and some will be reluctant to eat or go out to toilet because of the effect. Owners should not be alarmed, but be reassured that this is likely to herald a positive response to treatment. However, absence of sedation does not indicate a likely absence of response.

Clinical response

The clinical response to acupuncture is variable. There may be no response to the first treatment: this may be because the animal is not a responder, or because the treatment 'dose' was not strong enough; or because there was a brief response that was not recognised; or because one treatment is simply not enough for that individual. In these cases the stimulation in the second treatment could be more robust, as long as the patient can tolerate it, or trigger points may need to be targeted more directly, depending from where the worst of the pain (if pain is being treated) is judged to be coming.

There may be a worsening of the signs after the first treatment. The owner may report that the patient seems stiffer or sorer than before. This indicates that greater numbers of C fibres than A delta fibres have been inadvertently stimulated or that trigger points have been needled rather too vigorously. Owners should be warned that such an aggravation of signs may occur and may last several days, but that it usually indicates that the patient is a responder. The treatment should be modified next time to use either less stimulation, briefer needling times, finer needles or, if the problem appears after each session, all three. Owners should be advised that they can use an increased dose of the animal's current painkiller, if the clinician considers it safe to do so and if the patient is currently receiving a maintenance dose. The owner must be reassured that the condition has not been made worse and that no damage has been done.

There may be an improvement after the first treatment. The 'classical' response is an improvement in signs that may start from between day one of treatment to day three after treatment (this improvement is of course delayed if aggravation occurs first). The duration of improvement may be a few hours to a few days, but then usually the signs return to the level at the first treatment. After the next treatment the improvement lasts longer and is usually maintained; thereafter each treatment has a cumulative effect (Figure 10.4).

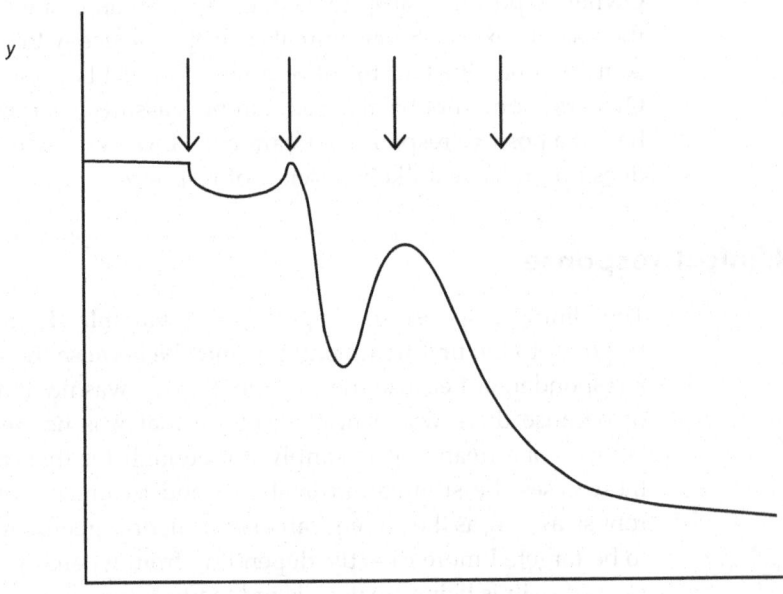

Figure 10.4 The classical response where y is the severity of signs and x is time. The arrows indicate each treatment.

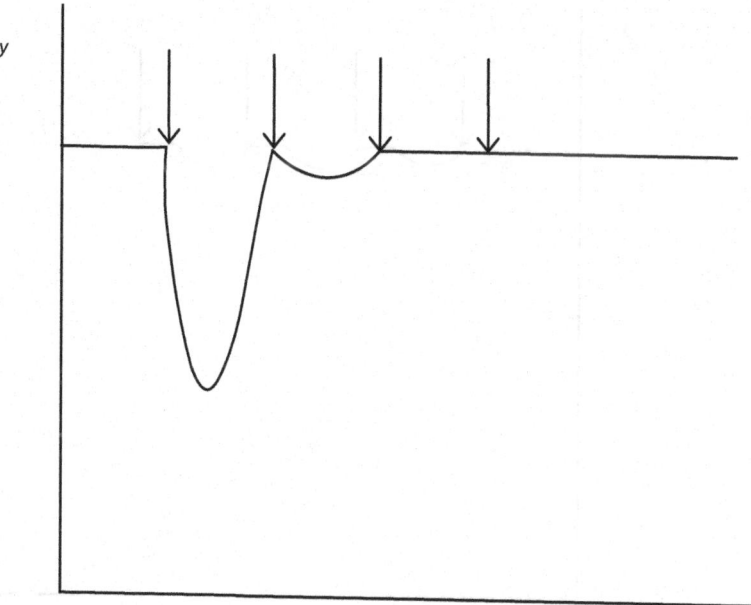

Figure 10.5 The so-called 'placebo' response. After the first treatment there is a dramatic improvement, but after the second treatment the improvement is not so marked and thereafter there is no response. The *y* axis represents severity of signs, the *x* axis time and the arrows each treatment.

Occasionally, a patient will improve dramatically after the first treatment and never deteriorate; in fact it can be difficult to know whether they should really be treated again at all. In practice, and so long as each treatment does not cause the signs to reappear, then a short course of three or four treatments could be completed and the owner told to return only when signs reappear. An apparent placebo effect also occurs occasionally (Figure 10.5).

Sometimes, it can be difficult to maintain a long-lasting response in patients (Figure 10.6). This may be for a variety of reasons, each of which should be considered by the clinician:

(1) There may be a particular behaviour that is maintaining the pain: for example, a horse may be continuing to jump when its conformation or an injury predisposes it to further soft-tissue trauma. A dog with osteoarthritic elbows and active triceps trigger points may be a compulsive digger; the pain of its behaviour only being apparent when the behaviour (and the adrenaline) has stopped.

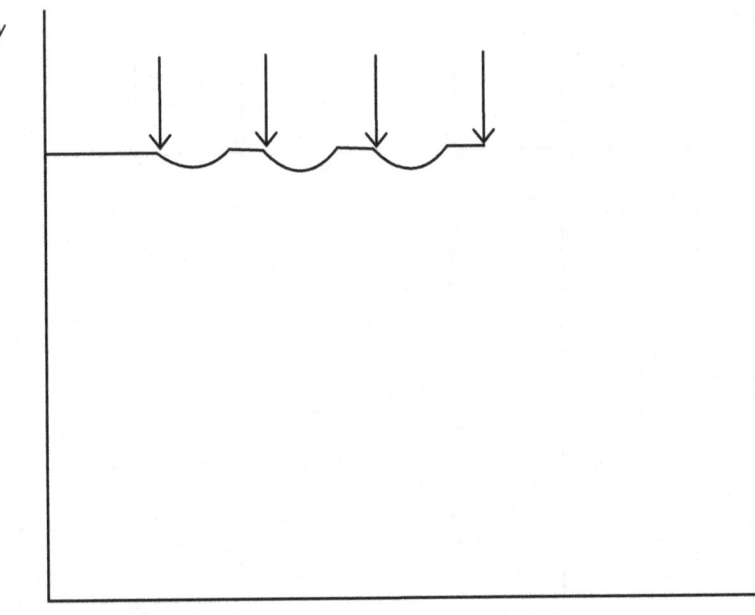

Figure 10.6 The unsustained reponse. There is a positive response after each treatment but there is no cumulative improvement. The y axis represents severity of signs, the x axis time and the arrows each treatment.

(2) The patient has a progressive condition such as malignancy or even osteoarthritis. The pain of end stage, non-functional joints is difficult to control by any means other than salvage surgery. A review of one's diagnosis and a check that no concurrent other disease process is occurring (such as hypothyroidism) is indicated by failing to maintain a response in a patient whose presented condition should respond to acupuncture.

(3) Some patients just seem to respond for a short period of time (a few days or a week) only, without any other obvious reason. Electroacupuncture may give a longer-lasting effect or other techniques may be needed to help alleviate pain if frequent acupuncture is impractical for the owner.

CONSIDERATIONS ON RUNNING A CLINIC

It is worth reiterating here that only a veterinary surgeon can legally administer acupuncture to an animal. It is not legal for a physiotherapist or any other practitioner, however well trained, to practise acupuncture, even 'under veterinary supervision'.

Themed clinics

Companion animal practitioners are familiar with the concept of clinics run on a particular 'theme', e.g. obesity or geriatric clinics. Whether such a clinic fits into the general scheme of the practice is obviously up to the individual practitioner and practice to decide. However the following points may be useful to consider.

Running a separate clinic for acupuncture and pain management

This approach has some practical advantages. Time slots can be tailored to fit individual acupuncture consultations rather than trying to fit in with regular appointment times. It may be more acceptable to the clients to see that these sessions are priced differently from regular consultations; for the practice the time involved can thereby be justified. If such a concept still exists in modern practice, the use of 'dead time' (pause for hollow laughter) in between surgeries could maximise the use of consulting rooms during non-consulting times and allow for staggered consultations in more than one room. Some practitioners like the whole idea of these clinics being something apart from the usual appointment routine and regard these separate clinics as 'time out' from conventional practice. While this may be the case, one must always bear in mind that it is not time out from being a clinician.

Practising acupuncture within usual consulting times

This may be practical and workable if appointment slots can be flexible, if other rooms are available and if a veterinary nurse is available for supervision. The initial work-up and examination will need a longer consultation, but if this has already been completed and a brief exam for tender points and trigger points that are still present and active is all that is needed, then treatment could be carried out within normal surgery time.

The initial consultation

It is important not to underestimate the time it will take to collect a full history and physically examine the animal, especially if the animal has been referred from another practice.

Clinicians should leave enough time to explain to the client what they are going to do and how the animal is likely to react and respond to needling. It can be useful to have a pre-printed leaflet explaining briefly how acupuncture works, possible side effects and responses to treatment. The owner can either have and read the leaflet beforehand, so that they arrive with questions ready; or they can take it away afterwards. Most owners request an explanation of how acupuncture works and this can take time unless using the briefest of explanations such as 'it works through the nervous system'. This is correct, but unlikely to satisfy many clients and may sound a little dismissive. Owners also need to understand how they and the clinician are going to measure a response in their pet, in other words, what outcome measures will they use to judge a response. Prognosis, frequency of treatments, changes in medication, in exercise regime and in diet also need to be discussed.

The initial consultation is often the only occasion that the owners have had to talk through their worries about their pet's condition, how much pain it may be experiencing and what they will do if acupuncture does not work (it will be a last resort in some cases; in fact most cases at the start of one's acupuncture career). Giving them time and listening to their concerns and expectations is important. Owners who feel positive about their pet's condition may well have an effect on the animal's demeanour, behaviour and pain perception (via neurotransmitter and humoral changes).

Bear in mind that some animals will be more active during treatment than others, so do not rely on being able to leave the consultation room during the treatment period. It is unfair and irresponsible to expect owners to cope with animals who are becoming distressed or restive, have lost a needle or two or are moving about excessively. It will sometimes occur that animals will find some of the needles painful and try to remove them with their mouths. *All needles should be counted* in at the beginning of treatment and out at the end.

Subsequent treatments

These can be shorter than the initial consultation, but it should be remembered that most clinical conditions change with time and re-examination is necessary both to assess progress and to identify those changes.

Parallel treatments

Running a clinic with two or more patients being treated simultaneously is likely to make more economic sense, but the factors discussed above should be borne in mind. Owners like to feel that they have the undivided attention of their clinician and a 'conveyor belt' feel is soon likely to be counter-productive. However, as long as the system is explained to them and sufficient time given to listen, these problems are not insurmountable.

Continuity

Once an acupuncture treatment has been started, regular weekly treatments are most likely to give the best results. This means that considerations of holidays and other time away need to take into account the stages of the various patients in their treatment regimes. It is difficult to expect owners to commit to bringing their pet for regular treatments if the clinician is frequently unavailable. With increasing numbers of veterinarians becoming competent in acupuncture, it is worthwhile contacting neighbouring practices or locum vets who practise acupuncture and may cover absences.

FARM ANIMAL AND EQUINE PRACTICE

From a practical standpoint, it is likely that acupuncture on the larger domestic species will be carried out during a visit to the stables or farm. It may be necessary to sedate some horses, so time should be allowed for this and supervision for the recovering animal available. An equine hospital may well be able to run a clinic if sufficient clients can be organised, but the same general considerations should be given to timing and supervision as outlined above.

Transport and liability

Consideration should be given to any immediate reactions by the horse to acupuncture treatment, especially on the first occasion, if it is going to be loaded and transported after treatment. From a legal standpoint, although sedation is unlikely to be so profound as to make the horse dangerously unsteady during transport, it would be better to avoid any perceived associations between needling and untoward events on the journey home. For this reason, it may be better to carry out the first treatment at the stables and observe the reaction to treatment before deciding to treat at the clinic; or to have stabling at the clinic where the horse can be observed to have recovered or to be normal before reloading.

Substrate

Bear in mind the substrate if carrying out acupuncture treatment in stables: needles are easily lost in straw and shavings; it is often better to treat in a bare stable or outside. If needles are lost it should be advised that the stable be cleaned out completely.

Safety of handlers and clinician during needling

One cannot predict an animal's response to needling; there may still be a response to deep needling or needling of trigger points even under sedation. The animal should therefore be as well restrained as for any other procedure.

Effects on group behaviour

It is advisable to leave the animal to recover in a stable before turning out, even if it has not been sedated, unless it will become unduly distressed by being separated from its companions even for a short period. Bear in mind that temporary changes in sedation, mood and pain perception can alter an animal's perception of threat and status and could potentially change group dynamics.

REFERENCES

1. Yanagihara M, Fujii T, Wakamatu N, Ishizaki H, Takehara T, Nawate K. Silicone granuloma on the entry points of acupuncture, venepuncture and surgical needles. *J Cutan Pathol* 2000;27(6):301–5.
2. Slovis NM, Watson JL, Affolter VK, Stannard AA. Injection site eosinophilic granulomas and collagenolysis in 3 horses. *J Vet Int Med* 1999;13(6):606–12.
3. Eriksson SV, Lundeberg T, Lundeberg S. Interaction of diazepam and naloxone on acupuncture induced pain relief. *Am J Chin Med* 1991;19(1):1–7.
4. Xu S, Pan Y, Xu S, Mo W, Cao X, He L. Synergism between metoclopramide and electroacupuncture analgesia. *Acupunct Electrother Res* 1983;14:103–13.
5. Kho HG, Eiijk RJR, Kapteijns WMMJ, van Egmond J. Acupuncture and transcutaneous stimulation analgesia in comparison with moderate-dose fentanyl anaesthesia in major surgery. Clinical efficacy and influence on morbidity and recovery. *Anaesthesia* 1991;46(2):129–35.
6. Lagerweij E, Nelis PC. The twitch in horses: a variant of acupuncture. *Science* 1984;225:1172–74.

7. Le Bars D, Dickenson AH, Besson J-H. Diffuse Noxious Inhibitory Controls (DNIC). Effects on dorsal horn convergent neurons in the rat. *Pain* 1979;6:283–304.

8. Chung JM, Lee KH, Hori Y, Endo K, Willis WD. Factors influencing peripheral nerve stimulation produced inhibition of primate spinothalamic tract cells. *Pain* 1984;19:277–93.

9. Campbell A. Methods of acupuncture. In: Filshie J, White A, editors. *Medical Acupuncture: A Western Scientific Approach*. Edinburgh: Churchill Livingstone; 1998. pp. 19–32.

10. Han JS, Ding XZ, Fan SG. Cholecystokinin octapeptide (CCK8) antagonism to electroacupuncture analgesia and a possible role in electroacupuncture tolerance. *Pain* 1986;27:101–15.

Electroacupuncture and related techniques

11

ELECTROACUPUNCTURE AND ACUPUNCTURE ANALGESIA

Aside from the accounts of 1835 of passing galvanic currents through acupuncture needles as described in Chapter 2, electroacupuncture is a modern phenomenon[1]. It was developed in China in the 1930s at a time when manual acupuncture was being used to induce analgesia for surgery because anaesthetic drugs were expensive and not readily available.

While the low intensity stimulation achieved by manual stimulation of the needles appeared to be effective, or at least effective enough to complete surgery, it did require a lot of input and constant stimulation from one or more acupuncturists. In order to reduce the number of acupuncturists required per procedure, increase efficiency and free up some elbow room for the surgeons, stimulation of needles by an electrical impulse generator was developed. This was termed electroacupuncture and the early machines used low frequencies of around 2–15 Hz because they were mimicking the frequency of stimulation achieved by manual acupuncture.

Parameters

Voltage and resistance

The electroacupuncture machine must generate sufficient voltage to overcome the electrical resistance of the tissues; the current that is delivered must be sufficient to depolarise the nerves. This current is dependent on the nerve diameter, but is in the region of 20 mA

(Reference 2). In comparison with transcutaneous electrical nerve stimulation, or TENS, which will be discussed in the next section, the electrical current required from electroacupuncture devices to depolarise nerves can be generated from a lower voltage because the skin's resistance is bypassed and Ohm's law applies:

$$V = IR$$

where V is voltage, I current and R resistance.

TENS uses pads applied to the skin and must therefore overcome the skin's resistance. Most electroacupuncture machines operate at 9 V.

Current and intensity of stimulation

The current required to induce analgesia must be strong enough to stimulate the A delta fibres (Type II and III afferents in muscle) and high intensity electroacupuncture is better at producing pain relief in chronic conditions than low intensity stimulation[3]. In practical terms this means that we try to deliver the highest intensity stimulation that our animal patients will tolerate.

Frequency of stimulation

Low frequency electroacupuncture of up to about 10 Hz releases beta-endorphins in the brain, while metenkephalins and dynorphins are released in the spinal cord[4,5]. The low frequency stimulation (2–4 Hz) of the early machines has been shown to be better at giving long-term relief of chronic low-back pain, although other kinds of pain may not respond so predictably to frequency[6,7].

Nausea appears to be controlled best at a frequency of 10–20 Hz and experimentally induced itch responds better to 80 Hz, while some wound healing experiments found no difference between low (2 Hz) and high (80 Hz) frequencies[8–10].

Therefore, the commonsense approach, in the absence of specific evidence for a given condition, is to stimulate at a range of frequencies so as to release as many of the neurotransmitters involved in the therapeutic effects of acupuncture as possible.

So, electroacupuncture is now carried out at a range of frequencies: at one extreme the 'low' or 'dispersed' rates of below 10 Hz are used and, at the other extreme, 'high' or 'dense' rates of over 100 Hz are used. It is usual for modern electroacupuncture apparatus to offer a combination of the two, the so-called 'dense–dispersed', in which the frequency automatically alternates between low and high every few seconds. This has the advantage of reducing accommodation of the nerve fibres to the stimulus as well as optimising the release of neurotransmitters.

Wave forms

Older electroacupuncture machines produced a spiked waveform when measured across an oscilloscope, but it is now accepted that a square wave is more efficient at depolarising the nerves at the lowest current. It was also suggested that a one-way flow of electrons from one electrode to another (i.e. between two needles in the body – essentially a fluid medium) produced a theoretical risk of electrolysis, causing a weakening of one of the needles through metal deposition in the tissues. Some of the older machines require the operator to reverse the polarity of the needles during treatment, thereby reversing the current, but modern machines generate a biphasic wave which produces no net flow of electricity and requires no additional adjustments during treatment (Figure. 11.1).

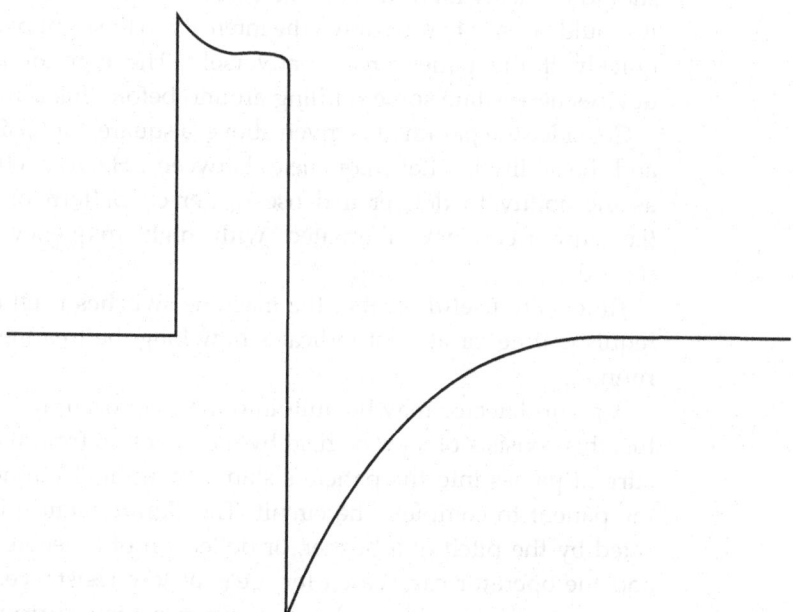

Figure 11.1 The square wave. Clearly this is not square beneath the line, but this represents the appearance of the wave when measured on an oscilloscope.

The pulse-width is usually fixed by the manufacturer of the machine at between 100 and 500 μsec (or 0.1 to 0.5 milliseconds). This is sufficiently long to stimulate nerves reliably, but not long enough to cause pain, as may happen with impulses over 500 μsec.

Features to look for in electroacupuncture machines for veterinary use

Consider the casing and sturdiness of the machine, especially if it is going to be used for large animal work or horses. Sudden movements of dogs have also been known to send machines crashing to the ground if they have been placed on a chair or table.

Consider the number of outlets: each outlet has a pair of leads, and the voltage across these leads can be increased by turning a dial, which is commonly labelled 'intensity'. Two needles can be stimulated per outlet. Some smaller machines have only two outlets, which will limit the number of needles stimulated at one time. Most machines have three or four outlets meaning that a maximum of eight needles can be stimulated.

Consider the clarity of design: it is important to have clearly marked dials that are large enough to be easily handled. Each dial should be easily identified with the outlet it controls; in other words it should be easy to turn down the intensity to the right pair of needles quickly if the patient reacts adversely. The ergonomics of some devices necessitate some fiddling around before this is achieved.

Consider the parameters given above: a square, biphasic waveform and the ability to alter frequencies between 2 Hz and 100 Hz, as well as the ability to deliver a dense–dispersed pattern of frequencies (i.e. low frequency alternated with high frequency every few seconds).

Timers are useful, so that the machine switches itself off after the requisite time, or at least indicates how long the treatment has been running.

A point-detector may be built into the electroacupuncture apparatus; this consists of a probe held by the operator, from which a small current passes into the patient's skin. A neutral electrode is held by the patient to complete the circuit. The skin resistance is then indicated by the pitch of a buzzer, or deflection of a needle on a meter, and the operator can search for areas of low resistance. In general, acupuncture points have lower resistance than surrounding skin, probably because of the presence of either sweat glands or superficial bundles of nerve fibres. But there are far more areas of low resistance than there are recognised acupuncture points, and most practitioners prefer to rely on the traditional anatomical descriptions.

Mechanism of action of electroacupuncture

In general, the mechanisms of action of electroacupuncture are the same as described for dry needling, but electroacupuncture appears to produce a greater range of neurotransmitters, which would logically be supposed to enhance the effects of manual acupuncture.

Indications for electroacupuncture

For the reasons described above, electroacupuncture is often regarded as being a stronger form of treatment than manual acupuncture and some practitioners use it widely when there has been no response to ordinary needling. The commonest indication is in the treatment of chronic pain and it may produce long-lasting relief. Electroacupuncture at 2 Hz has been shown to have a longer-lasting effect than either electroacupuncture at 80 Hz or manual needling in low-back pain[6]. It is also used for producing analgesia for surgery, and high frequency electroacupuncture may have a particular application in the treatment of drug withdrawal symptoms[11].

(1) Low frequency/high intensity (under the level of pain, but inducing muscle contractions) is useful in chronic conditions, since its effects are of long duration and cumulative (compared with TENS, which is not cumulative).
(2) High frequency/low intensity (pleasant vibration sense) induces production of dynorphins, and is short lasting, perhaps useful for acute or surgical pain[12].

In the veterinary species, the use of electroacupuncture is partly a function of the population treated, availability of electroacupuncture machines and the cooperation of the individual patient.

As a rule of thumb, it would be sensible to accustom the patient to dry needling for a few weekly sessions before embarking on electroacupuncture. In any case, it may be that the response to dry needling is satisfactory and electroacupuncture not necessary. The technique is more time-consuming than manual needling and because animals shift about more than human patients it is more awkward to fix and more difficult to maintain the needles in place if the animal is either not chemically sedated or does not become sedated by the treatment

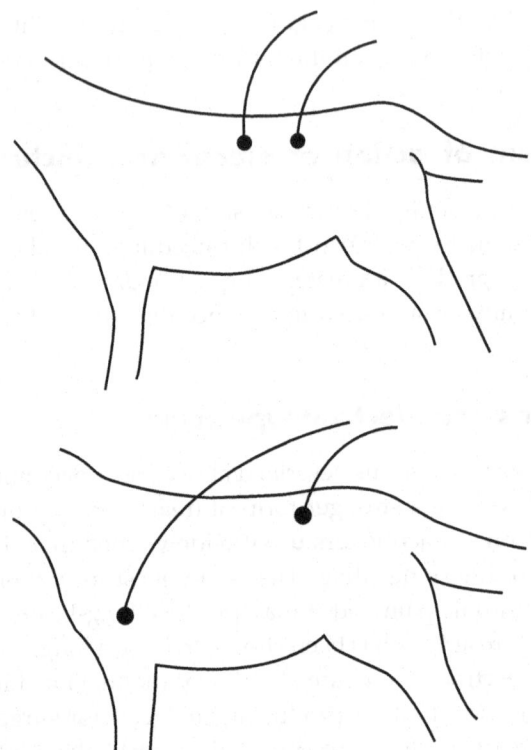

Figure 11.2 Paired needles in longissiumus muscles attached to an electroacupuncture machine, compared with one in the longissimus and one in infraspinatus.

itself. Having said this, most animals do accept electroacupuncture well; those that are sedated by manual needling appear to be more deeply sedated by this technique.

In general, it would be prudent to consider electroacupuncture in the following cases:

(1) If manual needling is effecting no response in the patient after three treatments and the clinician is sure of the diagnosis.
(2) If the treatment effect cannot be maintained, for example if the patient has to be treated weekly even after the initial course to maintain relief from clinical signs.
(3) If one is treating pain that is regarded to be particularly challenging, e.g. neuropathic pain or scar pain.
(4) If treating acute postsurgical pain or trying to achieve perioperative analgesia.

Clinical notes

(1) Choose points using the same principles of point selection as for manual needling.

(2) If the needles are far apart it is acceptable to pair needles close together, e.g. in the same muscle, rather than over large distances. For example it is more sensible to have two needles in longissimus muscle in the caudal lumbar area than one in longissimus muscle and one in infrapinatus muscle (Figure 11.2).

(3) Pair needles parallel to the spine rather than across it.

(4) Insert the needles deeply into muscle to a safe depth.

(5) Ensure all dials are set at zero and attach the clips to the needles ensuring that the metal clips are in contact with either the metal shaft of the needle (check that this shaft has not penetrated the tissue since the clips are not sterilised after use) or a metal handle. Note that some electroacupuncture machines can also be used as a TENS machine. On this setting the voltage is higher because the resistance is higher ($V = IR$) and switching on the machine with the TENS setting during electroacupuncture will result in considerable surprise and distress to the patient, owner and clinician.

(6) Increase the intensity to each pair of needles gradually, watching the patient's response. The aim is to reach the 'threshold of discomfort', which is when the patient starts to look a bit disturbed or uncomfortable by the stimulation. Turn the intensity to just below this.

(7) Muscle contractions may occur at higher frequencies and this is acceptable as long as the patient can tolerate it – and many do.

(8) After a few minutes it may be possible to turn the intensity up again.

(9) Treatment times are usually between five and fifteen minutes. Longer than 45 minutes is counterproductive because of the release of cholecystokinin (CCK-8), which antagonises some of the effects of acupuncture.

Contraindications and cautions

(1) Leads crossing the body, particularly thorax, head and neck are thought by some to be a hazard in human patients and it is not difficult to observe similar cautions in animals. (Note: in the USA the Food and Drugs Administration (FDA) prohibits the use of electroacupuncture on the head and neck in human patients, pre-

sumably because of a supposed resemblance to electroconvulsive therapy.)
(2) Theoretically, when used in the neck, electroacupuncture could induce hypotension and should be avoided, particularly in the vicinity of the carotid sinus.
(3) Electroacupuncture across the neck has been shown to suppress the function of a demand pacemaker in one human patient, although this incident was not associated with any clinical problem[13]. For the few canine patients fitted with pacemakers it would be as well to (a) discuss the use of electroacupuncture with the cardiologist, and (b) avoid stimulating in the area of the pacemaker.
(4) A history of epilepsy is regarded as a caution, perhaps more for veterinary legal reasons than any risk of inducing a convulsion.
(5) As with any needling, electroacupuncture should not be applied to broken or diseased skin.

TRANSCUTANEOUS ELECTRICAL NERVE STIMULATION (TENS)

Although this is used in some veterinary practices, it is mentioned here mainly because it is familiar to many veterinarians through their own use of the device or its use by a friend or relation. It would seem logical to apply the same technology to animals as has apparently afforded relief to many human patients.

However, the use of TENS would appear to be limited in the veterinary field because of its duration of action. For many people the effect of TENS wears off when the machine is switched off, so often the device is worn and switched on for much of the day. The electrode pads are in contact with the skin via a sticky gel and can be kept in place with the help of clothes, straps, belts or bandages if necessary. The machine itself is usually kept clipped on a belt or in a pocket. Clearly this is not a very practical arrangement for non-human patients and therefore the benefits are likely to be limited.

Mechanism of action of TENS – a contrast and comparison with electroacupuncture

Transcutaneous electrical nerve stimulation (TCNS or TENS) differs in that the electrodes are carbon-impregnated rubber pads, which are applied to the surface of the skin. TENS is therefore a portable system that is suitable for self-administration by the human patient.

TENS developed in the West in quite a different way from electroacupuncture: Melzack and Wall proposed the 'gate control theory' of pain to take account of a wide variety of different observations about pain[14]. One of these was that 'rubbing it better' can be effective, or in other words can 'close the gate' to pain signals. Wall and Sweet were the first to show that transcutaneous electrical impulses at a low intensity and high frequency (100 Hz) will relieve pain[15]. TENS has a thoroughly orthodox pedigree that puts it firmly in the conventional medical sphere and it is widely used in hospital pain clinics and labour wards.

TENS apparatus is now offering a range of continuous frequencies for the patient to try, most commonly between 40 and 150 Hz. There is also an intermittent variety called 'burst' in which short pulses of 100 Hz are delivered at the rate of one or two per second. A further refinement of this is the gradual increase of intensity through the burst, which is called 'modulated' or 'ramped', and is more comfortable for the patient.

More recently, apparatus has been designed to deliver the bursts to different electrodes in random order, which reduces the development of tolerance. And lastly, it has been found that some patients in whom ordinary TENS has been ineffective may respond to the burst form when given at high enough intensity to cause rhythmical muscle contractions. This is known as 'acupuncture-like' TENS because of the low frequency and muscle contractions that are typical of electroacupuncture[16].

LOW INTENSITY LASER THERAPY

Low intensity laser therapy or so-called 'laser acupuncture' merits a place in this section because of its wide use in the veterinary field and the frequent assumption that it is another form of acupuncture[17].

Acupuncture has been defined in many ways, but by the definition used for this book laser therapy is not acupuncture because there is no fine, solid needle used to penetrate the skin. However, it has been proposed by some that laser can achieve the same affects as acupuncture without the need for potentially painful or even risky needle penetration. The current evidence does not support this, although it does suggest that further study of the use of laser therapy, especially for pain in the veterinary species, and as an adjunct to other therapies including acupuncture, is potentially valuable.

Laser is an acronym for 'light amplification by the stimulated emission of radiation' and is often associated with the photothermal effects of high energy lasers used in surgery. The laser that is known as laser acupuncture is also known as low intensity laser therapy (LILT) or low level laser therapy (LLLT) and is athermic, i.e. there is no rise in temperature of the irradiated tissues.

Safety

There are health and safety issues associated with the use of lasers, including the use of goggles for clinician and patient (or owner) and the avoidance of irradiating eyes, fetus, any tumour or areas of haemorrhage, although specific risks for all of these have yet to be evaluated.

Parameters of treatment

Parameters of laser treatments vary, which makes assessing the therapy difficult. Efficacy of the treatment depends on the type of laser used, the tissue irradiated and the wavelength of the laser beam. The energy density delivered to the tissues determines whether the treatment is likely to be effective. It has been difficult to correlate dosages between humans and animals and the many trials that have been conducted give a wide range of irradiation parameters and measurement techniques, making it difficult to assess the overall effect of the therapy.

Mechanisms of action

In terms of wound healing, the mechanism is supposed to be of photomodulation, accelerating healing locally at a cellular level.

The mechanism behind the treatment of pain with laser is more problematic. Laser is extremely popular among many clinicians, veterinary and medical, but the evidence for its effect is variable. One of the biggest problems is that no convincing mechanism of action has been found. Most of the studies indicate that lasers may cause the release of neurotransmitters at sites distant from the stimulation sites; there is no evidence as yet of direct segmental competition at the dorsal horn as there is with needling. It may be that laser alters the perception of pain, rather than modifying the transmission of pain. If this is the case then it would seem sensible to use it alongside acupuncture rather than instead of it. However, until the trials use sufficient irradiation parameters it will remain difficult to assess the effects and efficacy of laser treatment for any species.

REFERENCES

1. Hamilton J. Account of a trial of acupuncture with galvanism, made by Dr W Stokes, a physician to the Meath Hospital. *The Dublin Journal* 1835.
2. White A. Electroacupuncture and acupuncture analgesia. In: Filshie J, White AR, editors. *Medical Acupuncture: A Western Scientific Approach.* Edinburgh: Churchill Livingstone; 1998. pp. 153–76.
3. Mao W, Ghia JN, Scott DS, Duncan GH, Gregg JM. High versus low intensity acupuncture analgesia for treatment of chronic pain: effects on platelet serotonin. *Pain* 8:331–42.
4. Han JS, Sun SL. Differential release of enkephalin and dynorphin by low and high frequency electroacupuncture in the central nervous system. *Acupunct Sci Int J* 1990;1:19–27.
5. Pomeranz B. Acupuncture research related to pain, drug addiction and nerve regeneration. In: Pomeranz B, Stux G, editors *Scientific Basis of Acupuncture.* Berlin: Springer-Verlag, pp. 35–52.
6. Thomas M, Lundberg T. Importance of modes of acupuncture in the treatment of chronic nociceptive low back pain. *Acta Anaesthesiol Scandi* 1994;38:63–9.
7. Lundeberg T, Eriksson S, Lundeberg S, Thomas M. Acupuncture and sensory thresholds. *Am J Chin Med* 1989;17(3–4):99–110.
8. Dundee JW, Ghaly RG, Bill KM, Chestnutt WN, Fitzpatrick KTJ, Lynas AGA. Effect of stimulation of the P6 antiemetic point on postoperative nausea and vomiting. *Br J Anaesth* 1989;63:612–18.
9. Belgrade MJ, Solomon LM, Lichter EA. Effect of acupuncture on experimentally induced itch. *Acta Derm Venereol (Stockh)* 1984;64:129–33.
10. Lundeberg T, Bondesson L, Thomas M. Effect of acupuncture on experimentally induced itch. *Br J Dermatol* 1987;117:771–7.
11. Marcus P. Acupuncture for the withdrawal of habituating substances. In: Filshie J, White AR, editors. *Medical Acupuncture: A Western Scientific Approach.* Edinburgh: Churchill Livingstone; 1998. pp. 361–74.
12. White A. Neurophysiology of acupuncture analgesia. In: Ernst E, White A, editors. *Acupuncture – A Scientific Appraisal.* Oxford: Butterworth Heinemann; 1999. pp. 60–92.
13. Fujiwara H, Taniguchi K, Takeuchi J, Ikezono E. The influence of low frequency acupuncture on a demand pacemaker. *Chest* 1980;78:96–7.
14. Melzack R, Wall PD. Pain mechanisms: a new theory. *Science* 1965; 150:971–9.
15. Wall PD, Sweet WH. Temporary abolition of pain in man. *Science* 1967; 155:108–9.

16. Filshie J, White AR, editors. *Medical Acupuncture: A Western Scientific Approach*. Edinburgh: Churchill Livingstone; 1998. pp. 177–92.
17. Baxter GD. *Therapeutic Lasers, Theory and Practice*. Edinburgh: Churchill Livingstone; 1994.

Index